Don't Let the
Bastards
Get You Down

D1561193

101 Strategies to Laugh Your Way
From Repudiation to Happiness

Mel Helitzer
Author of the Best-Selling *Comedy Writing Secrets*

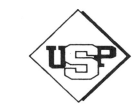

University Sports Press

Illustrations courtesy of:

The Cartoon Bank, a division of *The New Yorker Magazine*, Yonkers, NY, 10701

United Media Reprints for *Moderately Confused* by Jeff Stahler, 200 Madison Ave, New York, NY 10016

Universal Press Syndicate for *Ziggy* by Tom Wilson and Tom II, Kansas City, MO 64111

The Association of American Editorial Cartoonists, 3899 North Front Street, Harrisburg, PA 17110

The Cartoonist Group, PO Box 3163, Manhattan Beach, CA 90266

Funny Times, PO Box 18530, Cleveland Heights, OH 44118

King Features Association, Reed Brennan Media, Orlando, FL 32803

The Wall Street Journal, 200 Liberty St., New York, NY 10281

ISBN: 978-0-9630387-5-3

University Sports Press
P.O. Box 2315
Athens, Ohio 45701

Distributed by AtlasBooks,
A division of BookMasters, Inc.
30 Amberwood Parkway
Ashland, OH 44805

Special order through:
Amazon.com, BarnesandNoble.com,
Ingram, BookMasters or 800-Booklog

Library of Congress Cataloging in Publication Data: 2007902856

Foreword

I cannot remember one rejection that I have ever received in my entire life from my parents, brother, wives, children, lovers, business associates, university colleagues, or students. That, they tell me, is the first indication of Alzheimer's—or maturity.

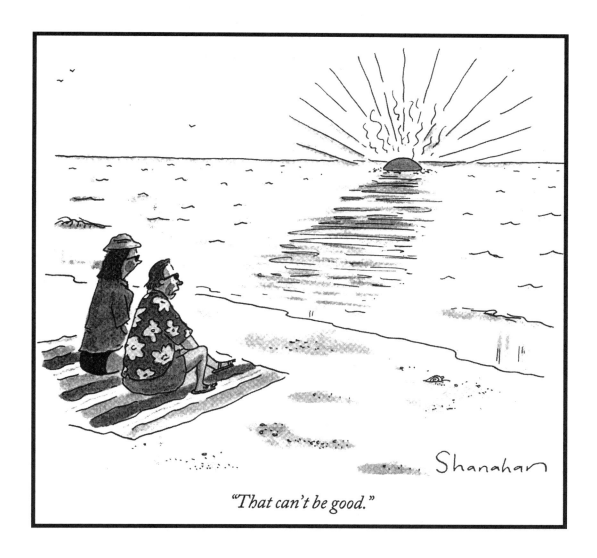

"That can't be good."

Other books by Mel Helitzer

The Youth Market 1970
The Associated Press Podium Humor Guide 1984
Comedy Techniques for Writers and Performers 1984
Comedy Writing Secrets 1986
The Dream Job: Sports Publicity, Promotion and Marketing 1992
Oh, Jackie: Her Father's Story 1999
It's Never Too Late to Plant a Tree: Your Guide to Never Retiring 2003

Contributing Writer

Executive Speeches 1993
Eisenhower and Mass Communication 1993
The Practice of Political Communication 1994
Light Dances: Illuminating Families With Love and Laughter 1997
How to Write Funny 2001

Video Tape

How to Write Humor 1987

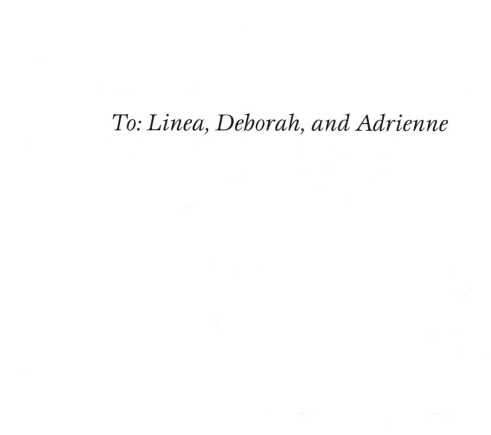

To: Linea, Deborah, and Adrienne

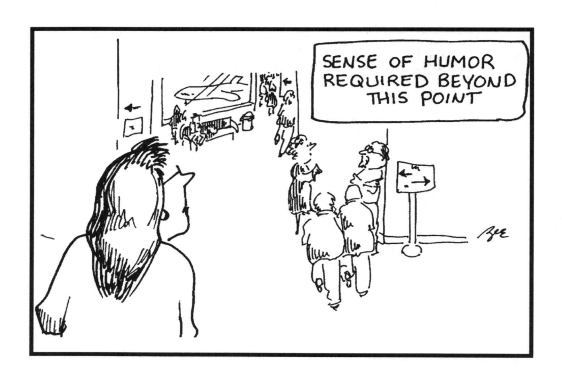

CONTENTS

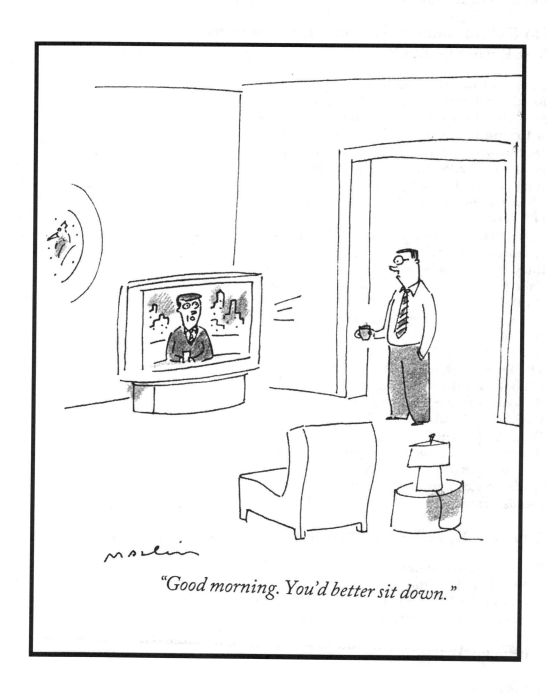

"Good morning. You'd better sit down."

Feel rejected? You're in good company.

Read what these celebrities did:

Christine Aguilera
Tim Allen
Pamela Anderson
Jennifer Aniston
Dina Arbus

Tyra Banks
Warren Beatty
Tony Bennett
Halle Berry
Erma Bombeck
George Bush

Michael Caine
Truman Capote
George Carlin
Hillary Clinton
Anderson Cooper
Sofia Coppola
Bill Cosby
Katie Couric
Norman Cousins
Marcia Cross
Billy Crystal
Mark Curry

Paula Deen
Robert DeNiro
Princess Diana
Joan Didion

Elizabeth Edwards
Sally Field
George Foreman
Michael J. Fox

Mahatma Gandhi

Salma Hayek
Hugh Hefner
Jennifer Hudson
Kate Hudson

Terri Irwin

Samuel L. Jackson
Elton John
Wynonna Judd
Lyndon Johnson

Jackie Kennedy
Bob Kerrey
Alicia Keys

Patti LaBelle
Shirley Lord
Joan Lunden

Howie Mandel
Ann-Margaret
Helen Mirren
Kate Moss
Eddie Murphy

Barack Obama
Clifford Odets
Lamar Odom
Kelly Osbourne

Sean Penn

Debbie Reynolds
Condoleezza Rice
Michael Richards
Jackie Robinson
Karl Rove
Beverly Sills
Alicia Silverstone
O.J. Simpson
Adlai Stevenson
Martha Stewart
Sharon Stone

Charlize Theron
Gene Tunney

Meredith Vieira

Mae West
Vanna White
Michelle Wie
Vanessa Williams
Oprah Winfrey

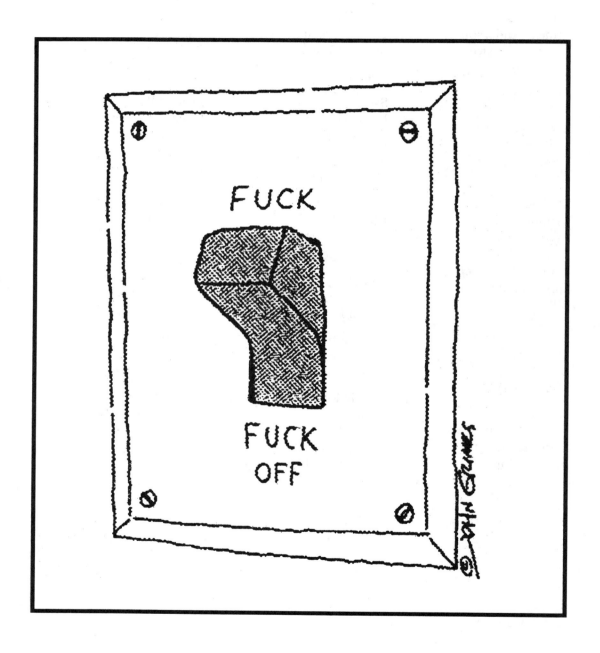

I Think Everyone Is Entitled to My Opinion

A comedian says funny things and a comic says things funny. In this book, I will prove that I am—a professor.

Rejection sucks. But it's not the end of the world. And the purpose of this book is to look at repudiation as one accepts pigeon droppings on a park statute. You can't stop it and you can't kill all the pigeons, but their doo-doo is no big deal and you can clean it up. The Japanese phrase *Mondai Nai* ("no problem") induces a positive feeling by encouraging you to spend less time on the problem and more time on the solution.

"I'd love to change the world, but I can't find a big enough diaper," said Myq Kaplan. Many colleagues, such as psychologist Mark Shatz, view repudiation more seriously, and sociologists such as Judy Pearson and Paul Nelson believe rejection occurs when others treat you in a manner that is inconsistent with your self-definition. Losses are teachable moments. And while the pain associated with any loss should not be minimized, there's a thin line between denial and humor as a motivator. But the theme of this book, which we will repeat over and over, is that it's O.K. to be pissed, and that a humor pill can reduce heartache pain, but you must always adjust to a new reality. In his best-selling book *Who Moved My Cheese?* whose thesis is that nothing gets better until *you* change, Spencer Johnson wrote: "The fastest way to change is to learn to laugh at your own folly—then you can let go and quickly move on."

Food for thought: This book, written in basic journalistic style, is a travel guide of 101 recommended rejection stops. It scrutinizes two analytical techniques: the first is that humor, although controversial as a text lubricant, is one of the most powerful communication devices in the world. That's why the text is accompanied by a library of cartoons, illustrations, quotable quotations, anecdotes, bits of esoteric information, and reformed clichés. At a university, it's not what's taught, but what's caught, so when we professors get our students' mouths open for laughter, we can slip in a little food for thought.

One size does not fit all: The second technique, like preparing a military campaign, is that no strategy can fit every battle. To be effective, this battle on rejection must include you as a commander. The 101 strategies can stop repudiation from metastasizing into a clinical depression, but only you can select the one or two that accurately cloak your situation. Now smile!

Mel Helitzer
Professor
Ohio University
Helitzer@ohio.edu

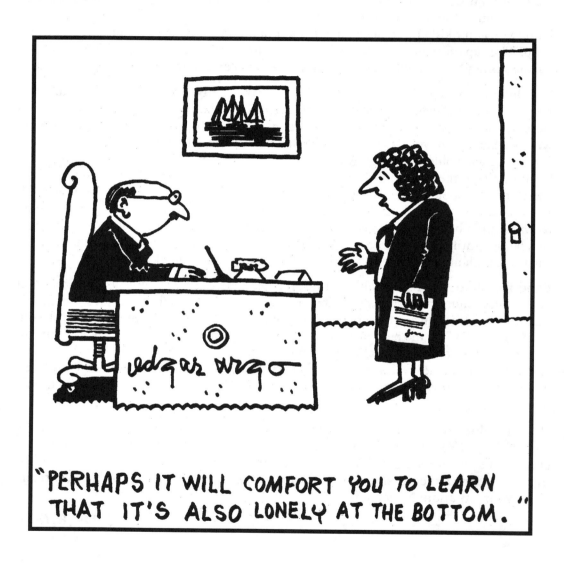

Rejection Is a Misnomer—
The Opposite of Woe Is Giddy-Up

Rejecting rejection: There are dozens of popular academic metaphors for rejection, such as a head of steam that has the potential to explode if not properly vented; or a closed door that can be opened if you can get a handle on it; or a ladder that can take you down or up depending on how you triumph over challenges; or the idea that rejection is not failure, but just one speed bump on the road of life; or the distinction between the words *anger* and *danger* depending on how well you manage the letter "D"—as in destruction. In truth, rejection is first a physical reaction. It is a punch in the stomach that can make you puke, and then, as time dictates, it can cause chronic diarrhea as it becomes a major pain in the ass. What it all translates to is that while negative action can cause unbelievable destruction, positive action can help make you a stronger person. So the next time rejection strikes, don't just stand there and fume, do something!

Heir bags: Rejection leads to anger, then to hate and—if not controlled—to depression—where you feel like a failure as a person. Rejection in children can result in stuttering. That's what happened to Van Gordon Sauter, who became president of CBS-TV only after he was able to overcome a childhood speech problem.

I've been sort of crabby lately. It's that time of the month again—when the rent's due.
—Margaret Smith

The light fantastic: "The word "no" is one of the shortest yet one of the most emotional words in our language. In personal development, it's one of the first words babies hear. Professional managers have recently noted that under-30 workers tend to be vulnerable (like crying in the office) when they are criticized. Career coaches blame it on the fact that so many were over-coddled as children and now, as grown-ups, suffer from an entitlement syndrome. "It's not O.K.," warns Robin Ryan. "Crying like a baby is a horrific career mistake."

When you're young, self-image is the way others see you. As you grow older, rejection comes from a sudden drop of anticipatory expectations. There are four generally acknowledged stages following rejection: (1) denial, (2) anger, (3) humiliation, and (4) self-blame. But with guidance, you can learn how to use rejection for future acceptance. Just because you're a victim doesn't mean you have to become a social outcast. This book is not for people who wish to find God, but for people who want God to find them.

There are three words guaranteed to humiliate any man: "Hold my purse."
—Francois Morency

You shall overcome: In mathematics, to turn a negative into a positive takes a formula. In life, the formula to turn a negative into an asset is called control. As with fire and water, if you can't learn to control the elements, they can be deadly. The optimist claims that if you're given a lemon, make lemonade. The pessimist says be realistic, don't open a lemonade stand until you've gotten a bushel and a license from the health department. There are those who say that hope is not a realistic alternative to action, but without hope there is rarely a spark for ignition. The Pete Seeger song "We Shall Overcome" keeps being used and used again as an anthem of hope for different movements. Taken from a 19th Century gospel song, the

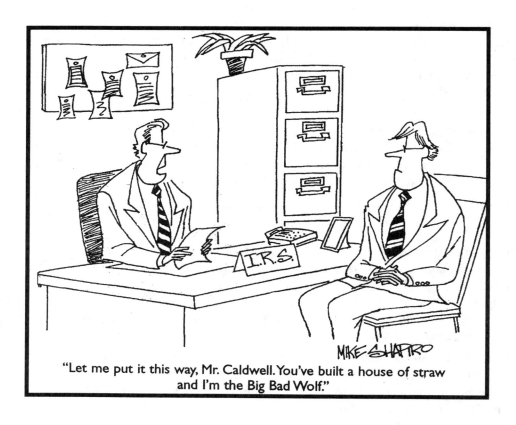

"Let me put it this way, Mr. Caldwell. You've built a house of straw and I'm the Big Bad Wolf."

words and melody have infused the Civil Rights Movement, were used by Chinese liberals at Tiananmen Square, played during the funerals at Columbine high school students, and were heard all day on TV during the 9/11 rescue efforts. Bruce Springsteen's version, retitled "You Shall Overcome," has given hope to thousands of children with leukemia.

Solutions are not the answer. **—President Richard Nixon**

Good grief: The dream of perfection as a mechanism, says Azriela Jaffe, never works. It only sounds heroic. But if you keep setting higher and higher goals, you will always feel frustrated, if not humbled. Lighten up! Just the fear of rejection destroys your self-confidence. Tim Wendel, who teaches writing at John Hopkins University, claims that the hardest thing for young people these days, who live in a world of instant gratification, is learning to be patient. They can rarely accommodate the pace that life fulfillment is a slow process.

The reasonable man adapts himself to the world. The unreasonable man persists in trying to adapt the world to him. Therefore, all progress depends upon the unreasonable man. **—George Bernard Shaw**

The Kinsey Report: It's a fact that most celebrated achievers failed in earlier ventures, but their persistence was rewarded. According to Joey Green, in his book *The Road to Success Is Paved with Failures,* the following actors were fired by their studios or producers: Marilyn Monroe, Barbra Streisand, Tom Cruise, Humphrey Bogart, Yul Brynner, Regis Philbin, Billy Crystal, Barbara Walters, Clint Eastwood, Lucille Ball, Bette Davis, and Steve McQueen. And Alfred Kinsey, whose research helped change America's sexual lifestyle, died believing he was a failure because his Rockefeller funding and Indiana University support were abruptly terminated.

Don't take the gas pipe: Ellen Pompeo is one of those celebrities who believe in the "better late than never" adage. Depressed by the death of her mother when she was only four, Ellen failed at every job she ever held as an adult. It wasn't until she was in her 30s that a fluke assignment turned her into the star of TV's *Grey's Anatomy*. "I don't regret being a late bloomer," she said. "Had this happened to me when I was younger, I would have made a real ass of myself." Recent celebrity biographies are replete with stories of current VIPs who came back from the "dead" when the media headlined their bad decisions.

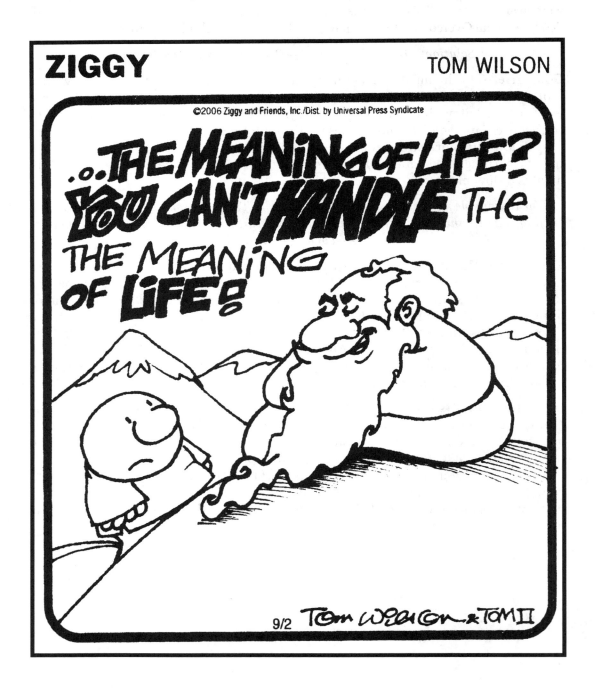

The Stress Mess—
The Three Most Frequent
Rejections

A true friend is someone who thinks you're a good egg, even if you're slightly cracked.

What it's cracked up to be: Despite rejections as a result of the shortage of money, poor credit score, or disheartening health problems, the three most devastating scenarios of rejection are:

(1) Rejection in love
(2) Rejection of a creative work
(3) You're fired!

Pass the peanuts: You haven't lived until you've encountered at least one. Rejection now covers sadness, depression, disappointment, dissatisfaction, in fact anything that impedes happiness, such as being complacent about a miserable marriage. Everyone has fear. Because, when you stop to think about it, fearless people are crazy. More importantly, don't die until you know what you can do about it!

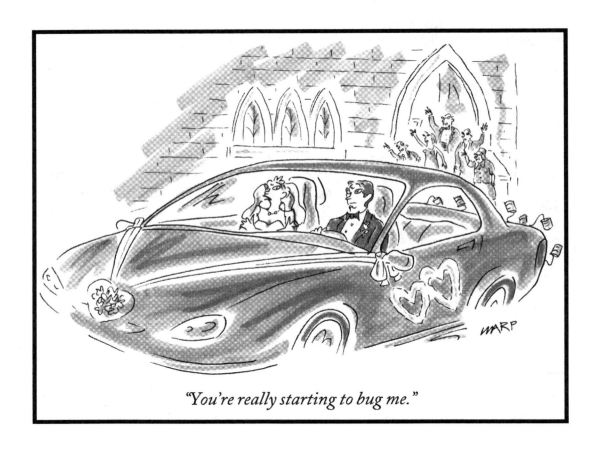

"You're really starting to bug me."

"I Feel Like Shit"—The Personal Split

It's hard to kiss any lips at night that have chewed your ass all day.

The ageless wonder: The only way to avoid feeling you've been punched in the gut by rejection in love is to fall in love with yourself. It's the oldest scenario in existence. A 16-year-old Narcissus did it watching his reflection on a river's waters. If you do it, you'll certainly have no rival.

*Love is like an hourglass, with the heart filling up as the brain empties.—**Jules Renard***

Love is just a four-letter word. Alienation or what might be more commonly called "loss of affection" doesn't start midway through a relationship. If we would admit the truth, it was inevitable because we felt it on the first or second date, and it was confirmed with the very first kiss or surely with the very first sexual experience.

*Girls are much more psychic than guys. They're the first to know if there's going to be any sex tonight and if you're going to be involved. —**Paul Rodriguez***

The wedding damn-er: If the doubt was there, then you played fantasy love when you should have stayed with fantasy football. There are a lot of reasons why one pushes to cement a permanent relationship even though our senses tell us it's wrong. Some of them are: (1) closure—a desperate need to take a lover because your eligible time is quickly running out, (2) the MRS degree—a petty need to satisfy a social standing, (3) fear of God—a religious need to have a husband for a pregnant woman, or (4) the trophy—riches, fame, or a handsome spouse blinds us. On the other hand, there is an increasing popularity toward lifetime single living—note Ralph Nader and Condoleezza Rice—and married couples now make up a minority of American households. "Now that I'm 40 years old, I will never marry again," said Halle Berry, "I've come to a place where I think two people can share their lives without the ring, without the piece of paper." "There's a mythology of marital superiority," claims Lee Reilly, author of *Women Living Single*. "Marriage does not transform miserable singles into blissfully married couples. Romance movies end too soon, without the full story where the princess is waiting for her prince to come—home."

Girl introducing one beau to another: "Albert, this is Edward. Edward, this is goodbye."

Corrective lenses: While our minds tell us the relationship won't work out, our hearts encourage us to charge forward, even though our senses fail to signal our inability to install corrective changes that are doomed to failure. What you first saw is what you're going to get. And the pain will keep you from the land of the rebound—jumping wholeheartedly into the next encounter.

*Most people think I'm a lesbian because of some bad sexual experience with a guy. Well, if that's all it took, the entire female population would be gay. —**Suzanne Westenhoefer***

Stray dogs: One of the biggest reasons for the increase in divorce is infidelity. So marriage counselors are urging couples to build trust upfront by acknowledging the possibility of cheating and heading it off at the pass. "If a partner does have an affair," says

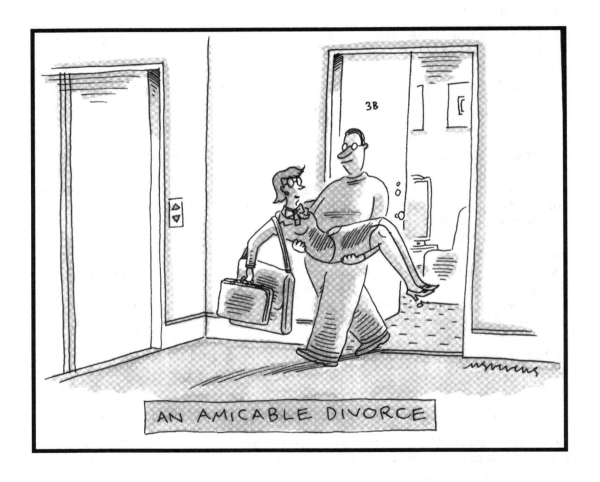

Barry McCarthy, a psychologist, "disclose it within 24 hours. It's the cover-up that has the most negative impact." According to Sue Shellenbarger of *The Wall Street Journal,* "As painful as self-disclosure appears to be, you can super-glue your marriage together by telling your spouse about an extramarital desire." Honestly!

Lost and unbound: However, when the relationship becomes so negative that splitsville becomes a destination, our personal recommendation is that you break up as quickly as possible. Time and effort will not heal it, although other important factors like children, religious taboo, and financial or community pressure may encourage one more try. This is most often a waste of time, and more importantly, a waste of mental, physical, and financial resources.

I've just learned that penguins are monogamous for life, which really doesn't surprise me, because they all look alike. It's not like they're going to meet a better-looking penguin some day.—Ellen DeGeneres.

There is no such thing as an "amicable divorce." Jan Collins and Jan Warner, Knight Ridder columnists, recommend the following tips: (1) the share of property is only half the battle, (2) consider interim estate planning like guardianship, to protect any children, (3) ensure that your documents will stand the test of time by covering all anticipated bases, and (4) consider including an arbitration provision to deal with changes of circumstances like emergencies.

A healthy state of mind. You can't settle a divorce if you slam shut your mind. Success comes despite anger not because of it. Benjamin Franklin wrote, "Anger is never without reason, but seldom with a good one." You need to develop a sense of well-being—"I'm better than this"—and to fight, but this time for peace. Be compassionate, not to your ex but to yourself. The starting point is letting go, putting out the fire before it gets too big.

Free love: After a reasonable adjustment period following a breakup, you're willing to try again. In was the 1960s anti-Vietnam youth, called the Woodstock generation, who contributed to the decline of connubial content by encouraging live-in partnership over ceremonial marriage. The latest manifestation of free love is the 100 or more free online dating services that can put you in touch with hundreds of different people from legitimate singles to illegitimate stalkers. Senders put out their personal profile, accompanied by the best self-portrait they've taken in 50 years, and wait for responses. It's recommended that you submit frequent batches of at least 20 before the lack of responses makes you feel so rejected that you start going back to bars, where at least the rejection is face to face.

My boyfriend and I broke up, even though we're still deeply in love. He wanted to get married and I didn't want him to. —Rita Rudner

One more time: According to Knight Ridder columnist Jeff Herring and others, here is what you need to look for and then let your mind, not your heart, confirm it:

(1) Marriage or a live-in relationship is about service. Even though you tested the relationship by living together for a long time, marriage changes things. Suddenly the fun of service becomes a requirement. Now you need to commit to not only

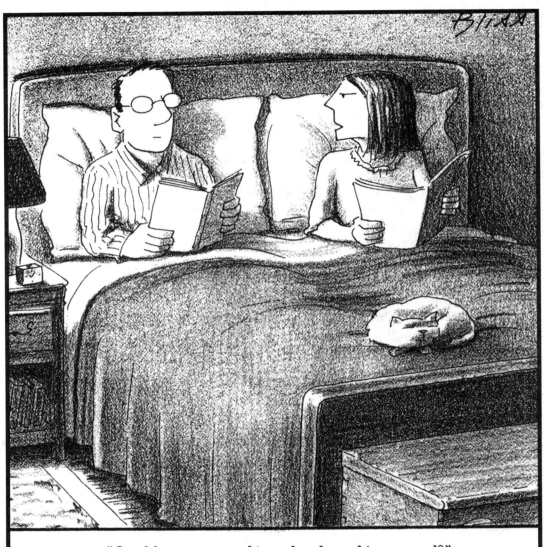

"Could you stop making that breathing sound?"

serving the other, but out-serving each other. You're being tested every day. Make only promises you can keep.

(2) Circle the wagons around the new family you've made. Place an imaginary boundary around the two of you. Friends and family might have a voice in how you're doing things, but you are the only two who have a vote.

(3) Accept that each of you has peculiarities. Learn how to react to differences so your poise isn't ruffled. Respect each other's traditions on ethics, political interests and how to handle religious observances, holidays and spiritual affiliation. Settle in advance the education of present or future children.

(4) Set up three separate bank accounts, one joint and one in each name, and agree on how each is to be funded.

(5) Make sure you agree on how to have fun, what it takes physically and financially to enjoy each other. It's important to continue to date each other long after you're living together. Say to each other every day "I love you," the three most important words in a long lasting relationship. Waiting until Valentine's Day and giving giant foam finger which says "You're number one" is no longer sufficient.

(6) Develop your own skills, and get a general agreement that the kind of work or activity you do outside the home is going to have unquestioned support from the other partner.

A sew-sew hobby: When Bryan Porter, a State of Ohio employee who supervises the high tension and emotional department of mental retardation, feels upset when programs do not go well, he comes home, changes clothes, and immediately sinks himself into house chores, plus motorcycle maintenance, computer art, sewing, gunsmithing, or collecting swords. His wife, Sandra, never asks about his office problems. She's happy that he's not only working off his anger but also getting overdue house improvements finished. You can't ask for a better solution than that, at least for a few days.

*My father was so cheap that every year he'd say, "I'm glad Christmas comes but once every other year." —**John Roy***

Shrink wrap: TV pin-up girl Pamela Anderson, partner in many publicized live-in relationships, has an unusual method for remembering how much each former boyfriend really cared about her. She saves their final emails. She said the messages confirm whether they really loved her or just made her think she was loved when she was not.

*You know that the relationship is over when little things start grating on your nerves. "Would you please stop that? That breathing in and out, it's so repetitive." —**Jerry Seinfeld***

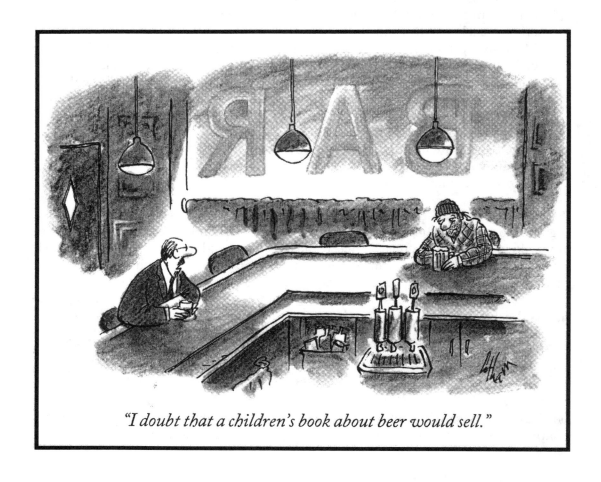

"*I doubt that a children's book about beer would sell.*"

The Slush Pile Rejection—Manuscripts, Applications and Grants

I loathe writing. On the other hand, I'm a great believer in money. —**S.J. Perelman**

Damnitol: "Rejection," wrote Carol Hoenig, "chips away at one's self-worth." But why anyone in this world is surprised when a manuscript is rejected is a greater surprise. The odds are so great against acceptance of a submitted proposal, whether it's for a publication prize or for grant writing, that you have to learn to embrace rejection, not personalize it. If you can't handle rejection, said Garrison Keillor, "get the money first, and then write."

Every journalist has a novel in him, which is an excellent place for it. —**J. Russell Lynes**

Mission almost impossible: There are 4,000 books published every week (more than 175,000 a year) and ten times as many submitted. We know of no author who has ever escaped getting rejected, even award-winning writers like Dr. Seuss, Sigmund Freud, Walt Whitman, Mark Twain, Charlotte Bronte, Jane Austen, John Grisham, and James Thurber. Many successful authors have gotten rejection slips ten times before a new work is accepted. Perseverance is necessary, because some stories need time to marinate. "My book *Looney Laws and Silly Statues* was rejected by a publisher," said writer Sheryl Lindsell-Roberts. "Five years later, on a hunch, I submitted the same manuscript to them again, and this time they accepted it. Was the content different? No, timing made the difference." Author and literary publicist Kathleen Miller Y'Barbo suggests that after allowing yourself a short cry, just admit that rejection was the publisher's bad luck in not being the one who published your book. The former president of Time-Warner Books said that rejecting the book *Tuesdays with Morrie,* a best seller for six years, was his biggest mistake in publishing, and the multi-million *Chicken Soup for the Soul* series was rejected by 35 publishers. Vladimir Nabokov's *Lolita* was rejected by publishers in Europe and America for years as "highly exciting smut." The first editor to read it did not think that adults who read it could escape jail sentences. Another recommended "that it be buried under a stone for a thousand years." So the relationship of who writes great stuff, who gets published, and who gets rejected defies logic because it is totally subjective.

You can't see the wind, either: In her book *Page After Page,* award winning author Heather Sellers claims that rejection is a way of life, part of the deal of being a writer. Instead of being pissed off, she advises, "Don't tense, don't complain and don't whine. Take your manuscript and send it out to the next name on your list. It should not spend one night in your house." She recommends her "3 R's for Rejection," a combination that includes (1) rerouting, (2) rewriting, and (3) research.

There are no dull subjects, there are only dull writers. —**H.L. Mencken**

Infernal affairs: Most writers try to find some glimmer of factual advice in every rejection letter. Most often, there is nothing more than a few words of courtesy. The best advice is to consider the editors as just a bunch of people who don't deserve the power they have. That's patently unfair, because editors are involved in a selection process, not a rejection

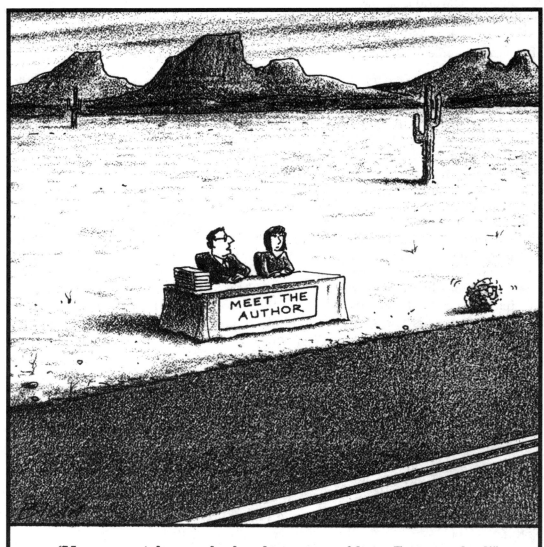

"*You are, without a doubt, <u>the</u> worst publicist I've ever had!*"

process, but it does promote an attitude that keeps you from becoming a serial killer. Another sound idea is to join a critique group that helps each other at weekly meetings with more advice, more eyes for checking and rechecking facts, and more shoulders to cry on.

Jackasspirin: After you've digested the rejection slip, toss it—no, on second thought, shred it so you're not tempted to look at it, or even paper your walls with letters that show your friends you're a writer whose material has been read by major publishers. Sellers claims her first book was rejected 17 times, and now it takes an average of ten submissions for a story of hers to be accepted. It is not unusual for a manuscript that was even paid for not to be published. Waiting time between submission mailing and reply may take as long as four months. Tony Carrrilo was a student at Arizona State when he applied for an opening as the student newspaper's cartoonist. The editors got tons of submissions and Carrilo's first samples got lost among the others. So he submitted again and not only got the college job but his cartoons also now appear in more than 100 newspapers nationwide. "Don't be afraid of rejection," he advises. "Too many people get that first rejection letter—or none at all—and think, 'O.K., that's it. I quit!' You can't quit. You have to toughen up and believe in your work."

A typo is not a blood type: Rejection slips keep you from being self-centered. And your envious friends appreciate the fact that you don't brag. But to keep their balance, rejected writers often practice writing retorts, the funnier the better. For example, the next time a publisher sends you a rejection slip that says "Your manuscript wasn't bad," write back and say, "It wasn't meant to be." When George Bernard Shaw received this telegram from a play producer, "Send manuscript. If good, will send check." Shaw wired back, "Send check. If good, will send manuscript."

Intervention: My daughter, Deborah L. Helitzer, ScD, is a professor and an assistant dean at the University of New Mexico School of Medicine. As a researcher, she has had success in securing millions of dollars in grants from governments, corporations, and multi-sized foundations. Her acceptance rate is about one in every three proposals, so she gets rejected often. "I don't think that success is a goal, just part of the journey, so I turn every rejection into a learning experience," she wrote. "I no longer write grants thinking they are going to be accepted the first time around. I write the first one the best I know how, but I am anxious to get them out so that I can get feedback on how to improve them. It works like a charm, and I'm much more emotionally balanced than when I expected every single grant request to be approved."

If you can't annoy someone, there's little point in writing. **—Kingsley Amis**

Magnificent possession: Even more onerous than grants are seedy rejection letters that doom applicants for admission to collegiate programs. Harvard turns down nine out of every ten students who apply, so 20,000 of the most talented high school seniors in the country received rejection letters this year. After posting a $100 application fee, candidates are very touchy about rejection letters that are unprofessional. Mitch Frye lists three major requirements that institutions should consider when mailing out rejection notices: (1) the rejection decision should be made quickly and the notice returned at a reasonable date, (2) it should be personalized, and (3) it should not be part of a mass email. Candidates are proud individuals, even if colleges have lumped them into the "many fine candidates" dumpster. In a 2006 film titled *Accepted,* a student

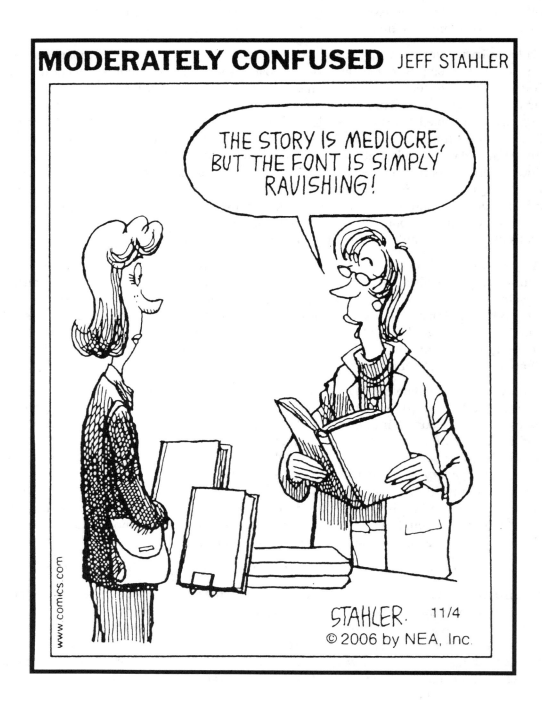

who had been rejected by every college to which he applied faked an acceptance letter from a fictional college. He fooled his parents and hundreds of other students who believed they had been accepted for admission.

For the record: By far the most quoted of all rejection slips is this one:

Your manuscript is both good and original. It's just that what's good is not original and what's original is not any good. **—Samuel Johnson**

Revenge: A former student, Mary Jo Crowley, a comedy writer, famous for discovering the Jewish dinosaur "OyhaveIgotsaurus," suffered through a long period of publisher rejections in her early years. Her antidote was this reply:

"I'm sorry to return your recent rejection letter. Frankly, I have received so many of them lately that I do not have need for any more at the present time. In addition, yours was curt, frigid, and uninformative. It was also not the best written. In the future, I recommend that you improve your communication skills if you wish to continue to be in a supervisory position. Good luck in the future. You're going to need it."

POD: With the growing success of print-on-demand (POD) publishing, one of the more popular ways to reject rejection is to self-publish your own material. It's no longer that difficult or expensive. One example is Matthew Diffee, a cartoonist, who published *The Rejection Collection: Cartoons You Never Saw, and Never Will See in The New Yorker*. He picked samples from thirty cartoonists who had received rejects from the country's most sophisticated literary magazine. It was of great delight to writers everywhere when an article by John Kenny appeared in the *New York Times* with a humorous portrayal of a fictional manuscript editor who unfortunately turned down J.K. Rowling's Harry Potter series, the greatest selling books outside of the Bible.

The Editor's Tale

"DID I have the chance to buy the first "Harry Potter" manuscript? Yes. Do I regret it? Not for a second.

"I remember the day I read it. It was Christmastime and I'd just returned from a longish luncheon at Le Cirque. I had the venison and rather a lot of the claret. I was celebrating because I'd almost been named editor of the year at our firm. Also, they'd forgotten to tell me where the company Christmas party was being held and I decided to hold my own. It had taken me longer to get back to the office, as I had difficulty determining east from west.

"When I did arrive, the office was empty. On my desk I saw a manila envelope. The cover letter was from an agent I'd never heard of. British. Said the enclosed manuscript was "the next great children's book," a 'Goodnight Moon' for preteens." I laughed. My father, who had also been a book editor before turning to taxidermy, had passed on "Goodnight Moon," and he and I often laughed at that.

"Did I mention that I have taken, at the chairman's and human resources department's urging, a much-needed sabbatical and am working at LeFrack's fish processing here in northern Maine as a scaler? I am.

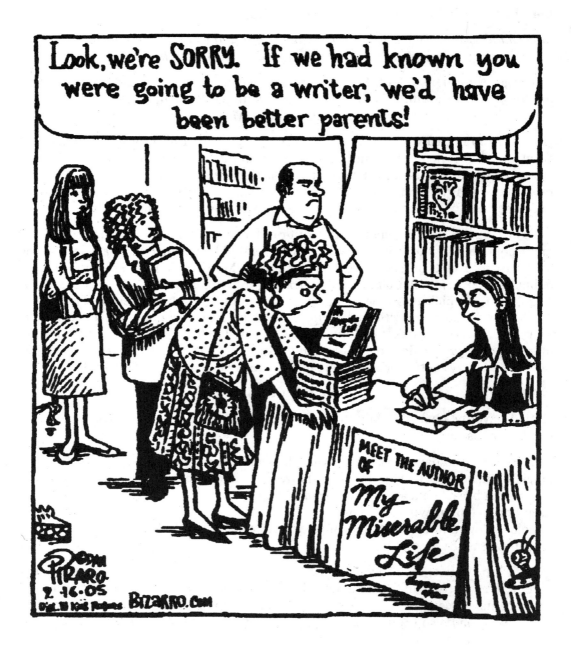

"It's funny to look back on that time. And, I might add, to look back without any regret. I've always thought myself a rather keen spotter of "the next big book." Certainly that was my reputation. I don't wish to boast, but I distinctly remember the day I signed N. Wizbicki for her manuscript "Spontaneity and How to Plan for It!" I remember it because earlier that day I had passed on Charles Frazier's "Cold Mountain." This was on the heels of "I Climbed Everest Without a Hat," to my mind a far superior book than either "Into Thin Air" or "The Perfect Storm," both of which I passed on.

"I used to have a cell phone but the court said that I am not allowed to now. Sitting across from me, at this very moment, is my colleague Rose, who works at the station next to mine cutting the heads off the fish and removing their intestinal tracts. Often I can smell nothing else for days.

"Where was I? I read the first few chapters of this so-called manuscript and, frankly, thought it drivel. February, perhaps March of the next year, I received a call from J. K. Rowling herself. She asked if I had had a chance to read her manuscript. I'm always embarrassed when fledgling writers get me on the phone. Most are sad, lonely people with no real means of income.

"I said I enjoyed her work a great deal, but that it didn't meet our needs at this time, the standard industry brush-off. There was a pause and I thought the line had gone dead when I heard laughing. "Mr. Wortham," she said with a light British accent. "I was calling as a courtesy, actually. To tell you that I sold the book. To Scholastic. For . . . " The line went dead. Or perhaps I passed out. I forget which.

"At lunch some time later I overheard our chief executive talking about the success of the Rowling book. So I happened to mention, with a chuckle, that we'd had a chance to buy it. Why is it that one remembers a long pause? "Chief?" I said, though to this day I don't know why, as no one called him that. "You what?" he asked, his voice trembling slightly. Much of the rest of that meeting is a blur. My wife left me. Did I mention that?"

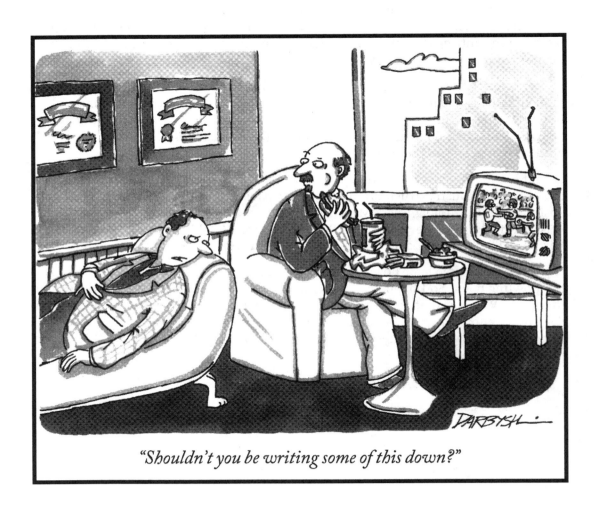

"Shouldn't you be writing some of this down?"

Writer's Block—When the Odds Are Against You

A word to the wise ain't necessary. It's the stupid ones who need the advice. —**Bill Cosby**

Life is a gamble: If you've written a book and are trying to find a publisher, your rate of success must first factor in the admission that every overnight success took years. James Joyce's blockbuster book *Dubliners* was rejected 22 times before being accepted. What if Joyce had quit after the 22nd rejection?

Catch-22: There are only about 1,000 respected literary agents who make a living only if their clients' manuscripts are accepted. They do not take on new clients in wholesale numbers. Many frustrated authors call this a *Catch-22* scenario. Agents don't want to take on unpublished authors, and only in rare instances will publishers consider even reading manuscripts by authors without an agent. Unsolicited manuscripts get relegated to the "slush pile," and most do not even get read, let alone returned.

Be an expert at something. There is always a market for someone who's the best, and even agents have their own subject specialties. Some agents have their best contacts with publishers who print historical novels, others with publishers that specialize in family sagas, or college textbooks, or cartoons, or biographies, or mysteries, or romance titles, or scientific material. The Writer's Digest Publishing Resource Directory has a roster of the largest literary agents, and recommends a web site—*www.agentquery.com*—that lists smaller agents by their area of interest.

Being small doesn't always have to say "I'm sorry." When submitting a query, some agents only want a brief letter, others request a query letter and a synopsis, and still others demand a sample chapter along with other introductory material. Practically all agents want to see an author's bio, the working title, a summary, the intended target audience, related and competitive titles that have previously been published, research on marketing opportunities, the present status of your manuscript, and any additional sales points.

Words to live by: Even getting a "letter to the editor" published in a major newspaper is a big gamble. The average big city daily, like the *Columbus (Ohio) Dispatch,* receives 12,000 letters a year, but prints only 2,200. That means roughly five out of six letters submitted see a big wastebasket. The reasons for deep-sixing your letter may have to do with (1) the number of letters received on that subject, (2) whether there are opposite opinions available so the paper can appear fair-minded, (3) eliminating name-calling, smut, or ethnic slurs that will not pass "go," (4) how often you have been published in that paper previously, and (5) whether your facts are authentic. The four main guidelines for crafting a successful letter: (1) keep it brief—50 to 1200 words, (2) make your point immediately plain—and one point is four times better than two, (3) be prudent—your words may be rebutted so don't attempt a hit and run attitude, and (4) check the publication's guidelines before submission.

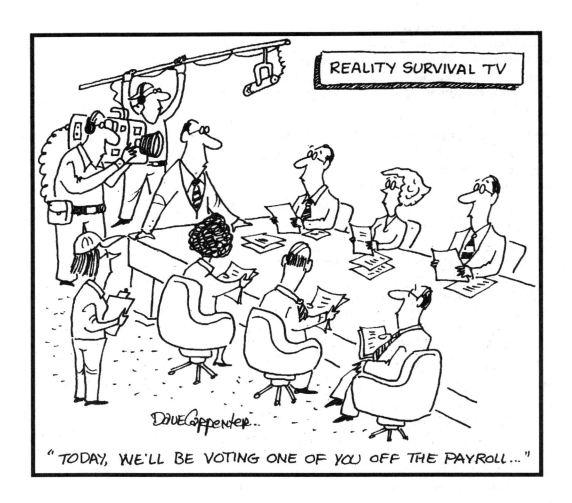

"You're Fired"—Getting Trumped

*A study said that one out of every four workers is angry at work. And the other three save it so they can share it with loved ones at home. —**Bill Maher***

Buzz off: Donald Trump didn't invent the *"You're fired!"* uppercut, but he did make it a buzz word for MBA students who are rarely taught to believe that this common rejection will ever happen to them. The first negative words that Vanna White encountered on TV had nothing to do with *Wheel of Fortune*; they came from Bob Barker, who fired her from *The Price is Right* because, he claimed, she spent too much time checking her hair in front of the studio monitor.

I always wanted to be somebody, but now I realize I should have been more specific. — ***Lily Tomlin***

Let my people go: Unemployment—whether it's called a layoff or a furlough—affects relationships in the family as well as the workplace. So be prepared to be fired, a condition that's a staple in business lexicon. It's not just employee deficiencies, but also reorganizations that come about from an industry paradigm shift, an unexpected product failure, mergers, acquisitions, downsizing, outsourcing, and public or government litigation.

*Having a job is a lot like sports. You have to practice every day, work out to stay in shape, study the greats. You hope to stay on the team, because it hurts to be cut. —**Sinbad***

A second chance: Some advisors claim that fighting for your lost job is a waste of time and valuable emotion. Don't believe it. Even when the decision to terminate you seems cast in stone, there have been enough examples of "I'll make improvements" to warrant speaking up and sharing your feeling. When Tara Conner, Miss USA, nearly lost her crown due to teen-age indiscretions, a teary-eyed plea to Donald Trump got her a reprieve and a short trip to rehab. "I have my flaws," she admitted. "I know it and now I know what to do." It also helps if you're a Miss Universe beauty. Meredith Vieira was fired twice during her long road to the top as a network news anchor. When she was 20, she was fired from a news job with a Providence TV station. Her dad said, "Do you believe you have value?" When Meredith said, "Of course," he answered, "Then how would anyone believe you unless you tell them." So the next day she marched back into the producer's office and said, "I'm going to prove you wrong." "O.K., I'm going to give you a second chance," he told her, "because this is the first time I've seen you have a backbone besides a pretty face." Many years later, as a news reporter for CBS, she got bounced by *60 Minutes* for demanding special hours to accommodate time with her first baby. But she went from there to *The View* and *Who Wants to be a Millionaire?* where she was so outstanding that NBC tapped her to replace Katie Couric on *Today Show*. Now that she has the prestige, the money, the whole thing, she adds, "At the end of the day, what counts is believing in yourself."

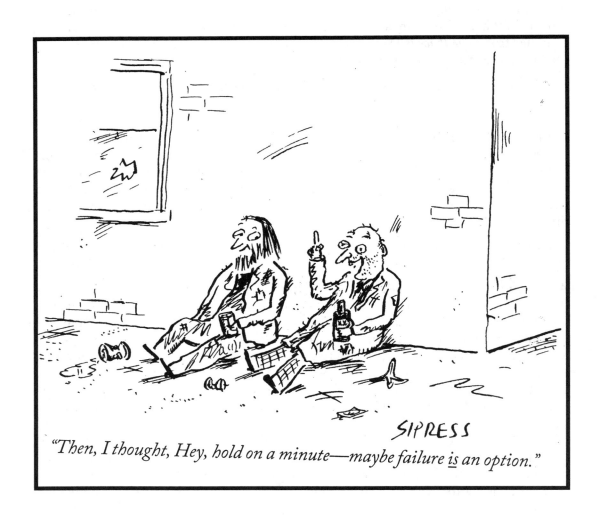

"Then, I thought, Hey, hold on a minute—maybe failure _is_ an option."

Do as I say: Even though many corporations have clear statements of acceptable ethical standards that employees must sign, ethical violations are more and more murky. There is nothing worse than leaders who preach high values but fail to follow their own advice or who set double standards. You will be constantly tested to stay true to such values because there are so many pressures to compromise them. For years textbooks have suggested that before making a major ethical decision, you should imagine how you would feel if your story were on the front page of *The New York Times*. Since that possibility is unlikely, it's more common these days to imagine your story being told by a whistle-blower to a grand jury. Then, if your conscience is not your guide, a parole officer could be.

Opening a can of words: We do not need celebrity executives running corporations into the ground for their own personal gain. Business needs more authentic leaders, but they are thwarted constantly by selection committee prejudices. For years, you would be rejected if you were not the right color, religion, or sex. Today, according to *Fortune* magazine, the average height of CEOs in their "500" list is 6 feet 1 inch, and a sizeable percentage are over 6 feet 3 inches tall. You must also have the ability to speak clearly without stammering. Poor speech habits damage an executive's career prospects.

Our topic today is déjà vu, so stop me if you've heard this before.

180 degrees: Another thing that has changed is a reversal of direction. Peter Drucker predicted that "the leader of the past knew how to tell, but the leader of the future must know how to listen." The courage to ask people's opinions and the discipline to follow up and actually do something has caused a revolution in management style. Testing of ideas with colleagues is more popular than instant decision-making. Rugged individualism is history. Today, no organization or society can survive for long without team leadership.

Noah's mark: MBA schools and corporate management are at odds over the need for executive loyalty. Graduates of many college programs are advised to change jobs every 18 months in the first few years, while CEOs are more aware that attrition is costly and they need to do more to retain promising interns.

*I had the meanest boss in the world. I would call in sick a lot, and I would say female problems. My boss didn't know I meant her. —**Wendy Liebman***

Dirty glancing: Personnel communication courses are another absentee blemish in the curriculum of most Harvard-like MBA programs. They spend more time on finance, accounting, corporate management, sales management, and mergers and acquisitions than they do on interpersonal communication. Yet more executives leave companies because of problems with their supervisors than they do because of compensation, job responsibilities, sexual discrimination, and promotion or approval credit. People don't quit companies, they quit people.

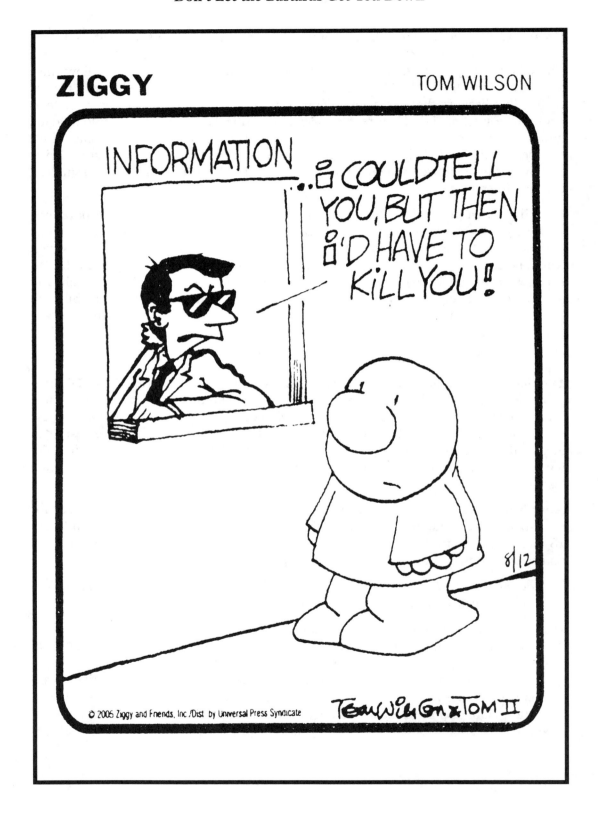

Getting in Control—
101 Rejection Strategies

The list starts here: In the following pages are 101 strategies for coping with rejection: avoiding it, overcoming it and even benefiting from it. According to Tim O'Brien of Knight Ridder, criticism is a basic form of rejection communication. While criticism is generally considered more destructive than helpful, you can grow from barbs directed at you. Just as workout training strengthens your muscles, managing rejection can strengthen your resolve. This book encourages the reader to put on the proper workout clothes and go to the rejection gym. A primary consideration is how you deal with critics, those difficult people whom Stephanie Rosenbloom defines as "jerks whose sour moods and explosive hysteria make our life miserable." Since you cannot defang them, it is better to put yourself in their shoes. For example, you might be the problem, not they. Then there are the Cassandras who predict doom for every project. The Talmud states that "we do not see the world as it is. We see the world as we are." So it may be better to listen to criticism carefully, and then ask your critic what he thinks the solution or next action should be. Someone once suggested that when a critic attacks a group of people, it may be actually good for the team. "If everyone really hates the person, it becomes the basis of social bonding for the rest of the group."

There are also the three C's of hardiness, a term defined by Madeline Uddo as the ability to shrug off stress by committing to *challenge* (an opportunity for growth), *commitment* (a purpose in what you do), and *control* (the ability to confront and influence the outcome).

Up and Adam: Nothing appears more resistant to rejection than the *challenge* through preparation. Since it is so obvious, the wonder is that it is so callously disregarded. The answer seems to be laziness. Samuel L. Jackson, whose films have taken in more money than those of any other actor in history, is obsessive about preparation for each role. He writes out and memorizes full fictional bios of each character he plays, including educational history, who his parents were, what he did, where he came from, what kinds of friends he has—all in order to act out even the tiniest barometric moments of character revelation.

The non-virgin queen: Helen Mirren, who won an Academy Award for portraying Elizabeth II in *The Queen,* was rejected for the part the first time she was considered because she had a reputation as "the sex queen of Stratford" for having been filmed naked in several films. But Mirren didn't allow her reputation and curvy figure from campaigning for "the best role I'll ever have in my life." Her *commitment* was to immerse herself in historical research. She studied the Queen's small bits of behavior, her gestures, her clipped cadence, and her dowdy getups. When she walked into the next audition "there was no way she wasn't going to get the part." She had become The Queen.

It is my belief that there are very few rejection events beyond our *control,* and the individual cases cover a wide range of practical experience and advice. Like prescription medicine, only a few may be relevant to you. And like theatrical rehearsals, the more frequently you practice them the more confident you will become.

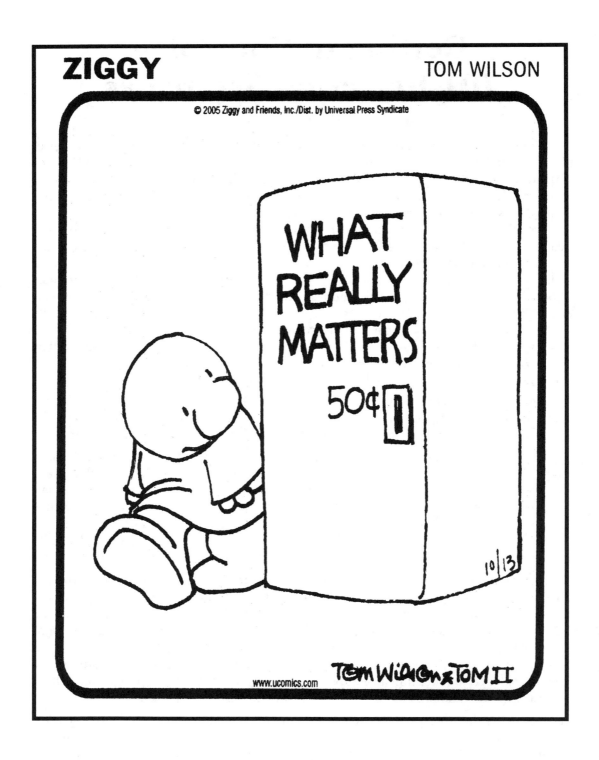

Stop Me If You Can—
12 Ways to Avoid Rejection

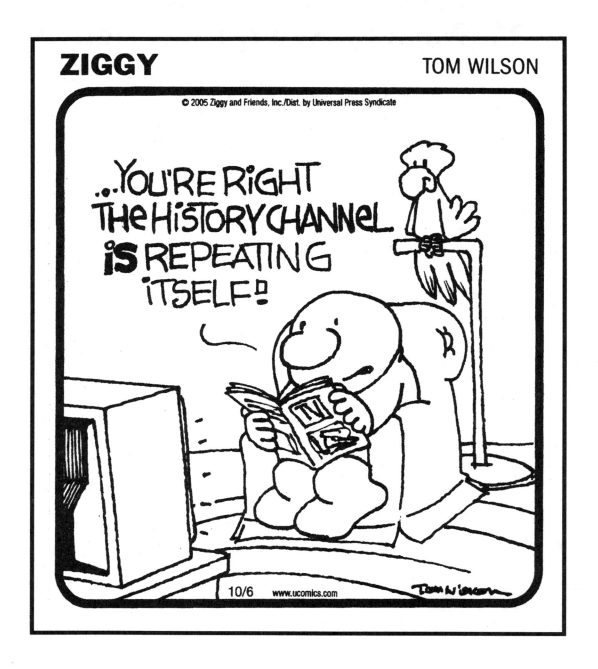

Profit From Another's Mistakes— Learning From History

Each time history repeats itself, the price goes up. —**Ronald Wright**

History lessened: Beat rejection to the punch. First admit your own constraints and frailties. "To be conscious that you are ignorant is a great step to knowledge," wrote Benjamin Disraeli. Therefore, you must never stop reading, you must never stop inquiring, and you must never stop listening, because you never want to stop learning. Seek books and articles to read, listen to tapes, and attend lectures, workshops, and classes. Study, read, and watch what others have done. You cannot survive if you do not know the past. Fool me twice, shame on me.

Never let the brain idle. An idle mind is the devil's workshop. And the devil's name is Alzheimer's. —**George Carlin**

History tells us that there are twenty top reasons for most rejections. Like a football coach's tape sessions, it's necessary to survey an opponent's plays in order to set your own deterrent game plan. And here's what humorists think about these rejection subjects:

(1) Prejudice: *Some people say all black people look alike. We call these people police.* —**Dave Chappelle**

(2) Over-estimating your ability: *I saw a commercial that said, "Kiss your hemorrhoids goodbye." Try as I might, I could never do that.* —**John Mendoza**

(3) Safety: *Screws fall out all the time. If the world is so imperfect, what makes you think you're not?* —**Mel Helitzer**

(4) Timing: *I never even believed in divorce until after I got married.* —**Diana Ford**

(5) The law: *Justice is not color blind. A white man will rob a pension fund of millions and go to jail for 12 months. A black man will rob a bank for a few thousand dollars, go to jail for 12 years.* —**Chris Rock**

(6) Appreciation: *You best appreciate water when the faucet is broken.* —**Keith Newman**

(7) Insufficient budget: *When I divorced I went through the various stages of grieving: anger, denial, and dancing around with my settlement check.* —**Maura Kennedy**

(8) Excess inventory: *When real people fall down in life, they get right back up and keep on walking, just like Bugs Bunny.* —**Carrie Bradshaw**

(9) Ignorance: *If stupidity got us into this mess, then why can't it get us out?* —**Will Rogers**

(10) Physical shortcomings: *Women claim that what they look for in a man is a sense of humor. Don't believe it. Who do you want removing your panties, Robert Redford or the Three Stooges?* —**Bruce Smirnoff**

(11) Self-inflicted wounds: *Life is all about choices, and generally there are two reasonable choices for every action. In order to succeed, your desire for success must be greater than your fear of failure.* —**Bill Cosby**

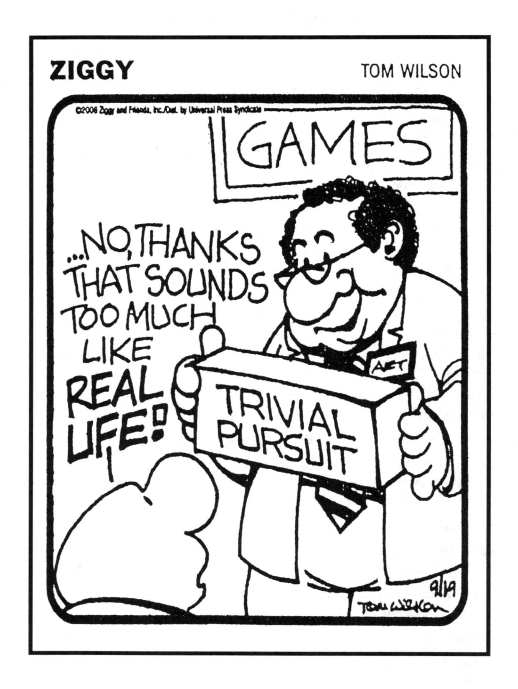

(12) Acts of God: *God works in mysterious ways, so don't try to anticipate his or her methods. "Thank God!" rather than "God, here's what I need."*

(13) Cost: *I was flattered when young co-eds started approaching me. Then I found out they only wanted me to buy them a few cases of beer. —**Mel Helitzer***

(14) Abuse: *If a man lies to you, don't get mad, get even. I once dated a guy who waited three months into our relationship before he told me he was married. I said, "Hey, don't worry about it. I used to be a man." —**Livia Squires***

(15) Community Mentality: *Labor Day is the day when we honor the most hardworking people in America. Let's take a moment to thank all those people by saying, "Gracias amigos!" —**Jay Leno***

(16) Need to Achieve Perfection: *You can fuck your way to the middle, but you've got to claw your way to the top. —**Sharon Stone***

(17) Resolution: *I have the same New Year's resolution every year. I decide to drink heavily. Because I know I can do it, it builds my self-esteem. —**Betsy Salkind***

(18) Politics: *The public just couldn't believe Bush knew what his administration was doing. Last November, he pardoned the Thanksgiving turkey, and the next day Vice-President Cheney shot it. —**Jay Leno***

(19) Immortality: *It's really important to maintain a positive attitude. It might not solve problems, but it will piss off enough people to make it worthwhile. —**Margot Black***

(20) Tradition: *Holiday traditions mean a lot to people, particularly people in retail. —**Michael Feldman***

You can overcome: Prepare for rejection every day, as hospitals and medical teams are lately preparing for an increasing number of disaster emergencies. If you're not prepared, you'll discover to your regret that catastrophes are not an eight-hour, nine-to-five possibility, but a callous 24-hour business. This means the odds are that a tragedy is three times more likely to happen when you least expect it. With riveting preparation comes confidence and self-esteem, because if you're not going to be part of the solution, then you'll be part of the problem. You'll be dependent on others who can step forward and ameliorate it.

> *I celebrated Thanksgiving in the traditional American way. I invited everyone in the neighborhood to my home. We had an enormous feast. And then I killed them and took their land. —**Jon Stewart***

Slow start, fast finish: Perhaps the most recurrent lesson from American history is that an early crash is not necessarily a lifetime derailment. If your last name is Roosevelt, Rockefeller, Kennedy, or Bush, it helps in politics even if your lack of syntax permits opponents to accuse you of having been born with a silver foot in your mouth. But being born dirt poor or even spending a few years in prison is only a temporary condition if you're willing to overcome it. It's even more difficult when you're the offspring of an unmarried Italian mother and an African-American father. At the age of 14, pop

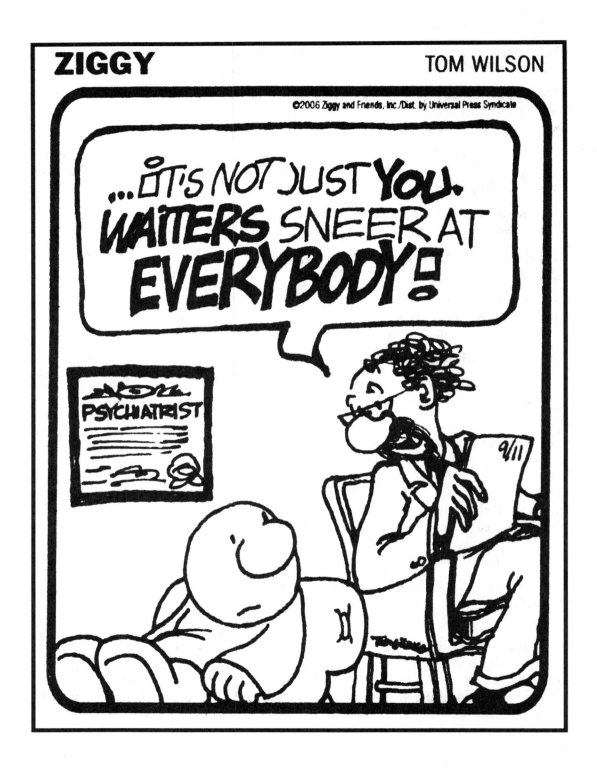

music star Alicia Keys lived in New York City's Hell's Kitchen, growing up around prostitutes, drug dealers, pimps, and strippers. "I was able to hang with people of any skin color, and any belief—the hardest, the baddest, and the worst." When her father disappeared one night, she turned to piano playing and writing music that people could really understand. "I just fit in everywhere," she said. "And I learned to honor myself, because no one will honor me if I don't respect myself. I learned not to be a quitter."

Queen for a day: Long before she was Hollywood royalty, actress Queen Latifah was Dana Owens, who cleaned toilets at a New Jersey Burger King. "But I was raised to not let anyone treat me poorly. When a manager was rude," she says, "I read him the riot act and quit. Sometimes when the crowd goes one way, your destiny may lie someplace else."

Pryor restraint: Few Americans have kicked off their life from a less fortuitous platform than Richard Pryor. His mother was a prostitute and he was raised in his grandmother's whorehouse. He atomized his anger and his constant depression by cradling a sharp wit, sifted through harsh and poetic imagination. One critic described Pryor's ability as "scaring us into laughing at his and our own demons, exorcising them through mass hyperventilation." He became so brilliantly funny he became an icon of American black humor.

Sing sing: Musicians Johnny Cash and David Crosby each spent time in prison waking up from being junkies. In 1927, Mae West was thrown in jail for ten days for refusing to stop portraying a low-grade character in a Broadway play she wrote. Bob Hope spent some of his youth in a reform school in Ohio. Tim Allen, whose father was killed by a drunk driver, tried to drown his tragedy by drinking and selling cocaine. He ended up serving two years in prison where he found out that he could turn his pain into humor.

Always be a first-rate version of yourself instead of a second-rate version of somebody else. —Judy Garland

History's take on love and family:

Not everyone can make it in America no matter how much effort and courage is available or displayed. Labels are still being stuck on people at first sight. It takes only 30 seconds to make a judgment that may last a lifetime. Trust is built in days.

I was asking my friend who has children, "What if I have a baby and I dedicate my life to it and it grows up to hate me. And it blames everything wrong with its life on me?" And my friend said, "What do you mean "if?" —Rita Rudner

You live three separate lives: one in public, one in private, and one in secret. The secret life is where your heart is, where your real motives are. The ultimate desires in your heart are things you wouldn't want to tell anyone, even your spouse. So create your own plan of life mantra—a sacred, verbal formula in a few words that you repeat over and over in meditation. It will keep you on track when all hell breaks loose—and it will.

The raging bull: Robert DeNiro received his greatest rejection on 9/11 when he watched the collapse of the Trade Center towers from his New York apartment ten blocks away. "Our neighborhood looked like a war zone," he reported. There were

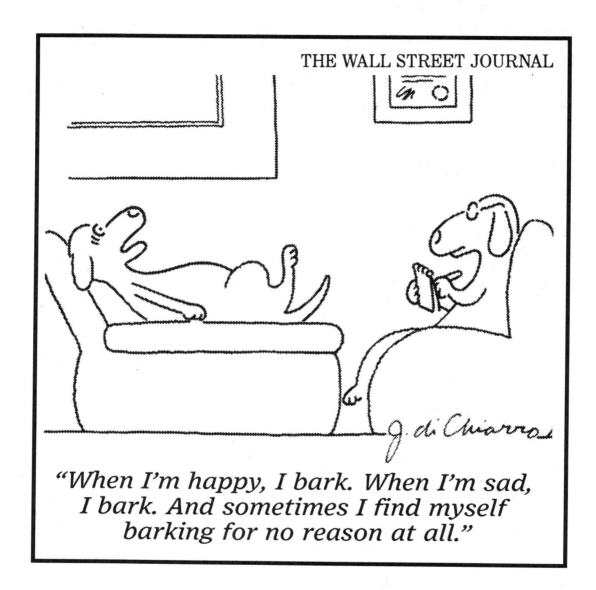

THE WALL STREET JOURNAL

"When I'm happy, I bark. When I'm sad, I bark. And sometimes I find myself barking for no reason at all."

emergency vehicles all over, there were police with machine guns and combat gear, there were helicopters buzzing over his head, constant sirens and a smell he has never been able to eliminate or forget. "We needed to give people, particularly the kids in the neighborhood, a new memory." So he co-founded the Tribeca Film Festival, a juried film competition, with panel discussions and an all-day family festival. Within a few years, the annual event had a profound healing and revitalizing effect on the Tribeca area pumping millions of dollars into the local economy by drawing more than 465,000 visitors to 800 screenings of films from 40 countries.

Love: Love may be the finest experience in the world, but most people despair of ever finding "true love." In fact, divorce is the single most frequent rejection in adult lives that discourages future intimate relationships. More than a million and a half Americans get divorced every year, and marriage breakups traumatize one in nine American adults. The more disastrous a relationship becomes, the more you see the pimples.

*I have a perfect record in marriage: three marriages, three divorces.—**Terry Bradshaw***

Eddie-Fying: Eddie Murphy is a master at jokes, but being involved in a thorny divorce was no joke, and Murphy was devastated. His basic humorous approach to womanizing worked against him in court and the eye of the public and media. He needed a new persona. His agent suggested another movie role, since the actor and stand-up comedian has starred in more sequels than any other performer in movie history. His idol has always been Elvis Presley, so Murphy campaigned for a role in the musical *Dreamgirls* that required him to do his own singing as well as play the part of a tragic character whose career is eclipsed by a female trio. "The part kept me honest," he claimed. "It took me to a different place emotionally and helped speed the divorce settlement. I saw the other side of the story."

As divorces become more frequent, so does the danger that the split will cause one of the parties to become a whistle blower to the IRS, the SEC, or to the FBI. These agencies are finding that rejected spouses have become a higher and higher source of serious criminal information. This was the case of Roger Blackwell, a famous Ohio State University professor and millionaire who got turned in by his ex-wife for insider trading.

*I married my wife three times and divorced her twice. She is a great housekeeper. After each divorce, she kept the house. —**Dick Linke***

There is no such thing as lasting love: "I'll love you forever," is a song lyric by Cole Porter but not a lifetime commitment. We understand last-minute broken engagements to avoid legal entanglements and condone the freedom to fail in love and marriage. By ducking out, we're increasingly reducing the self-blame of divorce ("If my wife—or husband—could see me now"), and increasing the popularity of live-in partnerships.

*It's important for people to know what you stand for. It's equally important that they know what you won't stand for. —**Mary Waldrip***

Family relationships between parent and child are more difficult than ever: Dr. Hiam Ginott once wrote," The reason grandparents and grandchildren get along so well is that they have a common enemy."

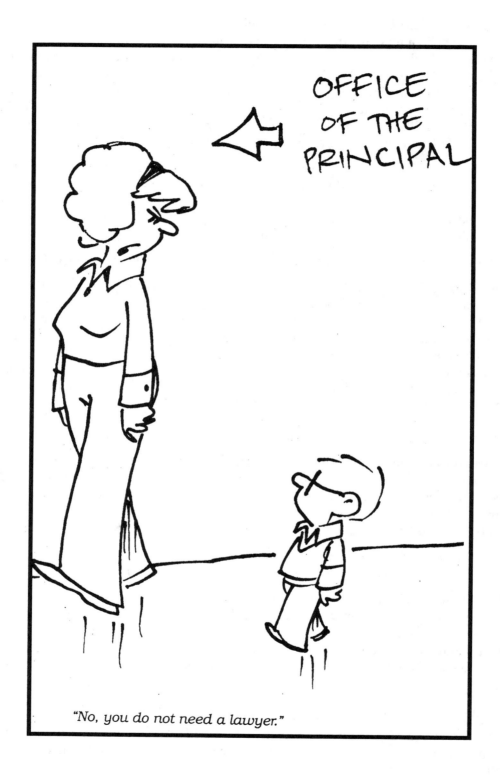

*My mother wants grandchildren. I said, "Mom, go for it." —**Sue Murphy***

Second time around: Rejection is increasing between children with stepparents when there are second marriages. Even more frequent are slights between brothers and sisters with different mental or physical qualities. And as soon as money becomes a factor, where there's a will there's a lawsuit.

*If you want to get rid of a man, I suggest on your next date you say, "I love you. I want to marry you. I want to have your children." Sometimes they leave skid marks. —**Rita Rudner***

Peer rejection among children can be caused by many factors—one of the most common is being gay or perceived as gay. Truman Capote claims he was beaten up often and as a result sought vengeance in his novels. Dr. Karen L. Bierman in her book *Peer Rejection* claims it is doubtful that the growing acts of violence on school grounds can be easily changed by adult instruction, exhortation, or reinforcement alone. "The best advice that child guidance counselors have agreed upon is that parents should watch out for antisocial behavior in their children." This simplistic exhortation will be about as effective as warning the public to report any suspicious looking people who might cause harm to their family. Hundreds of women turned in their husbands.

*My friend has a 16-month-old. The baby's crawling around and he has an accident in his diaper. And the mother comes over and says, "Isn't that adorable? Brandon made a gift for daddy." I'm thinking this guy must be real easy to shop for on Father's Day. —**Garry Shandling***

History's take on assorted subjects

Lighten up: Public complaints, such as a letter to the editor or an email poison-pen note, can get you into trouble because your whining stays in the recipient's mind long after the problem has been solved.

*Politics is supposed to be the second oldest profession. I've come to realize it bears a close resemblance to the first. —**Bob Orben***

Unrealistic exuberance: In politics today, the key word is honesty. And once you've learned to fake that, you're in. A politician who has not lost an election is as rare as steak tartar. Abraham Lincoln was one of the most quintessential losers of all time. At 23, he lost an election for the state legislature, at 26 he lost his girlfriend, at 27 he had a nervous breakdown, and at 28 he lost his business. At 34 he lost a Congressional election and at 45 and 49 he lost Senate elections. Despite repeated failures, he was elected President at 51. And 150 years after, he is still being rejected millions of times a day. Somebody minted his profile on a penny, and his one-cent copper in name only has become the most rejected coin in cash registers.

Grad to meet ya': Most universities require a Ph.D. degree to be a faculty member but never test how well the candidate can communicate or teach. Tenure is the most self-destructive honor a college can offer because it immediately minimizes the professor's dedication to accommodate a student's educational concerns.

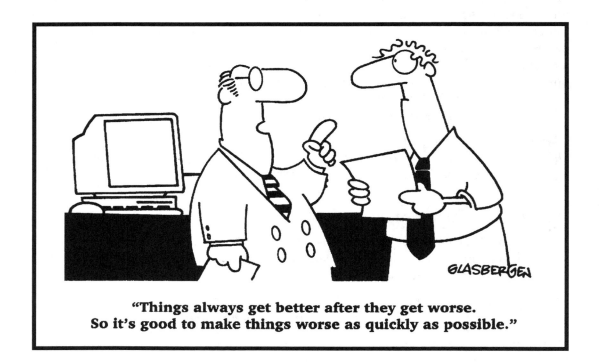

"Things always get better after they get worse.
So it's good to make things worse as quickly as possible."

A day without sunshine is like—you know—night! —**Steve Martin**

In sports: Records are so selective every competitor can claim some superlative sta-tistic: Babe Ruth's cumulative home run record was celebrated for more than fifty years, but the Bambino still holds the record for 1,330 strike outs. A more memorable rejection is the story of Buck O'Neil, the first black coach in major league baseball. In order for Negro players to get games with white pro teams, O'Neil in his youth toured with the Zulu Cannibal Giants and had to endure the indignity of playing in a grass skirt with his face daubed with war paint.

I think sports stars make great role models. Especially if you're thinking of a career in crime. —**Laura Kightlinger**

In the arts: There are three assignments necessary for every successful author: (1) skill-fully writing the book, (2) successfully marketing the book to a publisher, and (3) pro-moting the book to the public. In addition, personal relationships are increasingly important, but they should not be decisive. When Katie Couric was trying to decide whether to accept a CBS-TV offer to become the first female solo news anchor, a num-ber of her friends begged her to turn it down. But Couric rejected rejection. "At the end of the day," she philosophized, "it's just a job. It's not my entire life. I've experienced great loss (her husband and her sister both died of cancer) and each taught me that there are many important things to a rich life. If the job doesn't work out well, I'm confident there are other exciting things to do. You know when you're young, they give you tests that tell you what you should do when you grow up. Mine always came back that I should be a social worker."

Hard work pays off in the end, but laziness pays off now. —**Al Lubel**

A pain in the neck: There is a link between the anger of rejection and heart disease. Angry people are also more likely to sustain serious injuries. Anger, an emotion of ir-ritability that exists for self-preservation in a dangerous world, must be neutralized be-fore endorphins, that make you feel energized and calm, will enter your system. You're not alone. There are studies that claim 60 percent of anxiety-related personality traits are passed from parent to child. On the other hand, proper rejection techniques can help prolong your life. Anger is not just a natural instinct; it can be a positive one. Ac-cording to Alan Loy McGinnis, in his book *The Friendship Factor,* "Anyone who can not show true anger is inept at showing love as well."

He's the kind of friend who will always be there when he needs you. —**Adam Christing**

Attack rejection: Jerilyn Ross, a behavioral therapist, recommends making a three-pronged list of all the things that frustrate you. Look for recurring situations that set you off. "Once you know the triggers, then you can take steps to avoid them," says Ross. Next set goals for solving them, starting with the easiest. "Put yourself on a schedule," she claims, "whether it's tackling three issues a week or simply penciling in 30 minutes a day of quiet time to take stock of what's going on in your life."

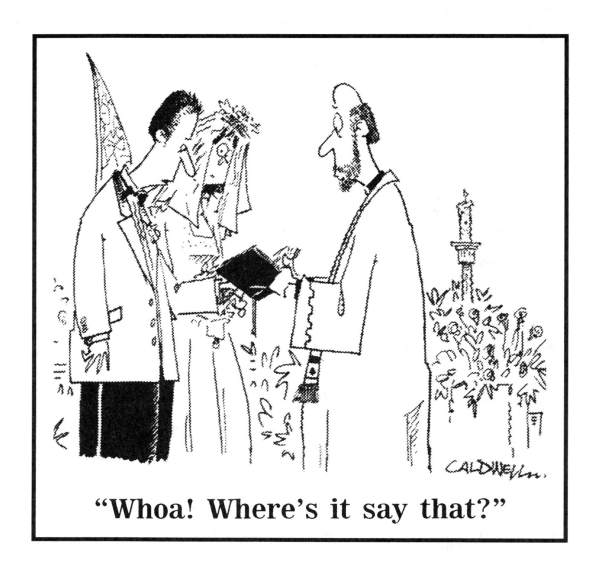

People are wired to focus on only a few things at a time. So focus on the few crucial goals that carry the most serious consequences. And don't become paranoid. An ancient survey once claimed that one in four people are so depressed by rejection that they become paranoid. You can test that. The next time you're with four close friends, look at them carefully. If they appear normal, and you think that you're the one paranoid, you've just passed the test.

I got to a traffic light, and it turned red. I shouted, "Why me?" —**Geoff Bolt**

Empty saddles: The feeling of rejection is reinforced by your habit of losing things, whether it's your car in a parking lot, or car keys, or hearing aids. Garrison Keillor's solution is worthwhile, "Don't change your clothes. Have one jacket with big pockets that you wear every day, no matter what, and keep your essentials in it. People will talk, but it'll save you six months of your lifetime and you'll get to read *David Copperfield*."

A brainy solution: Do men sense rejection as much as women? The answer is absolutely. That means yes! A man's emotional life is as complex as a woman's, but instead of obsessing over problems men do a better job of hiding emotion. Although both sexes cry, rage, shout and pout, they express their emotions differently. Josh Coleman, author of *The Lazy Husband,* claims men compartmentalize and intellectualize more. Experts say men's right and left brains are hard-wired differently, sort of a meandering country lane that prevents immediate access to feelings. Women, on the other hand—or other brain—have a left and right brain connection like an interstate highway. They rarely forget tiffs and will continue to stew over a slight the male has long since forgotten.

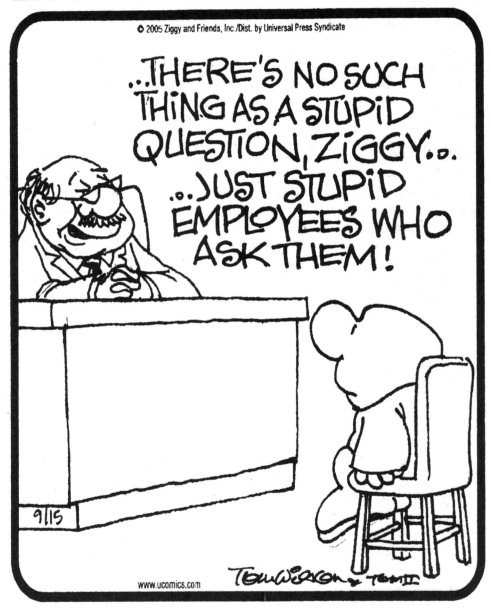

The Good, the Bad and the Ugly— Corporate Employment

A guy walks into the local welfare office, marches up to the counter and says, "I hate welfare and I don't think it's fair to be living off a government check. I'd really rather have a job." The social worker says, "Your timing is excellent. We just got a job offer from a wealthy man who needs a chauffeur for his beautiful, 20-year-old daughter. You'll drive his Mercedes, you'll be provided with a two-bedroom apartment on the estate, and he'll supply all of your clothes. Because of the long hours, meals will be provided. You'll be expected to escort her on her overseas holiday trips. And since she's a nymphomaniac, you'll have to satisfy all her sexual urges. The starting salary is $200,000 a year." The guy, wide-eyed, asks, "Are you bullshitting me?" The welfare worker says, "Yeah, but, you started it."

Train to win but plan to lose: If you play football, it's inevitable you're going to get knocked down. Whether sports are a perfect metaphor for business rejection is debatable, but the antidote for being beaten is not to dwell on defeat but to pick up the ball and play the next game. However, the antidote for a business rejection—and according to a Dilbert point of view things will always go wrong—comes from adequate preparation before the action, not after.

*My boss made me get glasses. I wasn't seeing things his way. —**Mark Klein***

Don't believe in business as usual. No business wants to be usual. It wants employees who are interesting, multidimensional and dynamic. If you are looking for employment in corporate America, let's pull back the covers of business myth and enumerate just a few of the bewildering array of the good, the bad, and the ugly that you need to know.

The Good:

*Most people work just hard enough not to get fired and they get paid just enough money not to quit. —**George Carlin***

Don't dread adversity. It challenges you to improve, and it's the way you will get stronger. You may not now be what you want to be or ought to be, but through rejection you will be thankful that you're not what you used to be.

*I lost my job. No, I didn't really lose my job. I know where my job is. It's just when I got there, there's this new guy doing it. I lost my girl, too. No I really didn't lose my girl. I know where she is, it's just that when I got there, there was a new guy doing it. —**Bobcat Goldthwaite***

It's the interview, stupid. Interviews may last a half-hour to an hour, but the first decision to hire you or pass is made in the first thirty seconds. The rest of the time is devoted to enhancing or changing that initial opinion.

A job resume is an exhibit not a selling tool: Nobody hires from a resume. It may help get you an interview, but more often it's a quick-read, leave-behind piece. Keep it short, no more than one page in length, in 10- to 12-point type. Cut the graphics and eliminate the colored paper stock. References and letters of recommendation should be on attached sheets. Do not list affiliations that ended with negative results. There

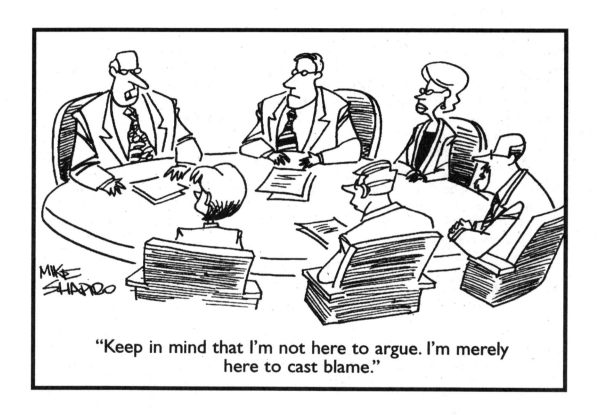

"Keep in mind that I'm not here to argue. I'm merely here to cast blame."

will be a void in your employment chronology, but there is no wisdom in pointing out scar tissue.

Boss to new employee, "You have nothing to fear except fear itself. And, of course, me!"

Sharp as a pin-stripe: Your character is on display with everything you wear, do, say and ask. In order of importance, the biggest turnoffs, according to human resource interviewers, are (1) poor grooming, (2) inappropriate attire, (3) a weak handshake, (4) piercings, and (5) visible tattoos. Worst interview technique: begging ("I really need a job."). How you dress sends a signal even before you say your first word. Business casual for both men and women is currently appropriate. For men, don't wear a Mickey Mouse tie even if you're interviewing with Disney, and for women with great legs, mini-skirts spell trouble even at a boutique ad agency. The old adages still work: you never get a second chance to make a good first impression, and you want to be remembered for what you say, not what you were wearing.

Best interview technique: First, understand that in many cases, you're looking to impress only one person at a time. Come bearing gifts—like a bright idea or a recommendation of how you will help improve the bottom line. When you hear the line, "People are our most important asset," don't believe it. Companies don't care about people, they care about results. Interviewers want to know how you communicate, how you listen and then respond. One of the common tricks human resource personnel use during an interview is to forewarn you that you may be rejected ("Unfortunately, you may be over-qualified for this job") just to test your character during a negative situation. Keep your cool and your sense of humor ("If I'm over-qualified, you'll be getting one heck of a bargain"). Just don't over-promise. There is a positive reaction called the "surprise machine," which comes into play when you've lowered management's expectations and then exceeded them.

Interviewers automatically distrust the veracity of those who claim they are "authorities." They now require everyone to supply evidence of their previous successes and awards. This comes from the cynicism of too much blogging and political spinning where even major news organizations, while trying to be factual, are also grinding out partisan axes. "No network or newspaper," according to William Raspberry of *The Washington Post*, "deserves to be taken seriously as seekers of truth."

When the captured outlaw begged for his life, the sheriff said, "I'll give you a chance. When I yell three, you draw and shoot." When the outlaw agreed, the sheriff said, "One. Two," then drew his gun and fired. "I thought you said, we draw on three," said the mortally wounded outlaw. "Three was your number," said the sheriff. "Mine was two."

A college degree has long been required for middle management applicants, and an MBA was desired. Yet, today, many firms are reading deeper into resumes to see if a high school start in real life business endeavors helped a potential CEO learn how to organize work efficiently and handle arduous schedules. Bill McDermott, CEO of SAP Americas, had several jobs simultaneously as a teenager. He worked as a supermarket busboy, as a delicatessen counterman, and as a food store owner. Today, he uses the

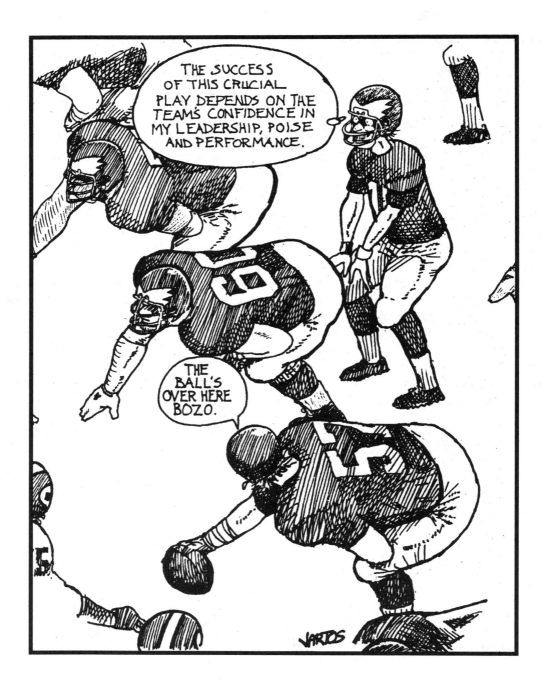

same marketing strategies he learned at the deli. "It's always the same," he predicted. "It's serving the customers so they want to keep coming back to you. Now I look for resourceful people who can figure out how to do a job better—and have fun doing it."

All salary decisions are negotiable. During your first job interview, you are involved in a razor's edge negotiation—it can cut two ways—and the best deal you will ever make with this company is the one you make at this juncture. Never be the first to name a figure—you will always lose. After discussion about the job's requirements, ask about the position's salary range, and then direct their focus to your accomplishments and then to your enthusiasm. The standard salary guide is that every employee whose work can be measurable must produce five to six times the salary amount to cover all benefits, support personnel, overhead, and profit.

If you can fool all the people some of the time—that may be enough.

Either oar: What if you've rejected a job and then you changed your mind? Don't be hesitant. Contact the employer as soon as possible. As long as the opening remains unfilled, no company will stand on pride and not reconsider a candidate who first impressed it with the skills and ability needed. Tell the company you've reconsidered because the other offers were asking you to decide too quickly. Now you realize that their offer was the opportunity that offers the greatest challenge—and you're ready for it. "The worst they can say is no," claims Perri Capell.

The Bad:

Holding on to your job may be more difficult than getting it. Most entry-level jobs are filled by college graduates who start out as interns. They expect college graduates to remain no more than two years before they start seeking career changes, but the costs of interviewing, training, and repairing new employee mistakes are rising so rapidly that management is demanding lower turnover. That's why more than 50 percent of all middle management jobs are filled internally by promotions or new assignments by present employees.

Downsizing: Don't expect fringe benefits in health insurance, stock options, maternity and sick leave, or even liberal expense accounts to last. They are on the chopping block of more companies struggling both with their bottom line and with surveillance by regulatory agencies. And when you ask to be excused from meetings in order to spend more time with your family, the company will remind you that they expect executives to think of the company as family.

You are either growing or shrinking. You can't know too much, so never stop learning about the vicissitudes of your market. Read publications such as *The Wall Street Journal, Business Week, Fortune, Forbes,* and *Leadership Excellence,* all of which are increasing their coverage of employee recruiting and human resource activities. Management is showering executives with more information on key issues, with review meetings and three-ring binders jammed with new material. There are now increased expectations that employees will do a lot of late night cramming. Work hard, work smart.

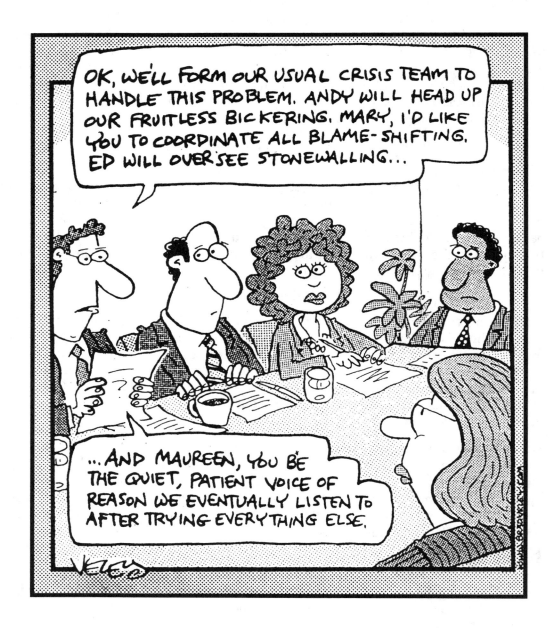

You must learn to be a leader in meetings. The ability to communicate and persuade has become mandatory. Management expects all its executives to write clearly, speak articulately, and inform concisely as well as accurately. Consumers do not trust those whom they can't immediately understand. It was common years ago for the CEO to make the decision after a comprehensive meeting. Today, however, with business increasingly complex, individual managers are being delegated with final planning responsibility.

The Ugly:

No Cinderella: James Joyce believed that mistakes are the portals of discovery, but in modern management, employees who make mistakes don't become researchers, they're fired. In business, there is no such thing as an accident. An accident is an example of someone who gambled and lost. The underlining corporate philosophy is that since you are collecting a paycheck for 100 percent of your work, you are also 100 percent responsible for all parts of your business life. This may be counter to real life, but forgiveness is not a business option.

Your personal life: can no longer have a direct impact on your business life. Most people mistakenly think it's the other way around. If your personal life is filled with turmoil, grief or pain, management will understand your difficulty in concentrating on even simple work assignments. Not now! If you can't grin and bear it, you can't even be a receptionist, hotel desk clerk, or even a waiter. It is your responsibility to work through your crisis. If you have a big problem, some companies are willing to offer help, but they demand that you be the one to suggest a practical solution that will not affect their bottom line. They are not interested in *how* things will be better. They want to know *when* things will be better.

Business life is a life of jeopardy: Treat your associates poorly and you will treat customers poorly. Just as whistle blowers are becoming more frequent, so too are embedded corporate spies among middle-executive ranks. They are assigned to watch and assess your daily actions. Expressing your anger, dislikes, intimacies, even grief openly can be dangerous as well as unpleasant. There are no bosom pals, and office sexual relationships can end up being more costly than a trip to the best massage parlor in town. Being paranoid in society can be unhealthy. Being paranoid in business can keep you from being fired.

There are some things in life where it's better to receive than to give, and massage is one of them. —Al Michaels

Forget about loyalty. Expecting a reward for over-achievement is a recipe for disappointment. The only work you owe your employer is if you have been paid a week in advance. And the only thing the employer owes you is an opportunity to prove every day that you are worth keeping.

Plan for the future: Research indicates that 80 percent of any company's successes are determined by only 20 percent of its employees. It is no longer brutal to remove the bottom 20 percent. According to a national poll, 77 percent of workers feel burnt out sometimes, and most of them claim a toxic boss is the reason.

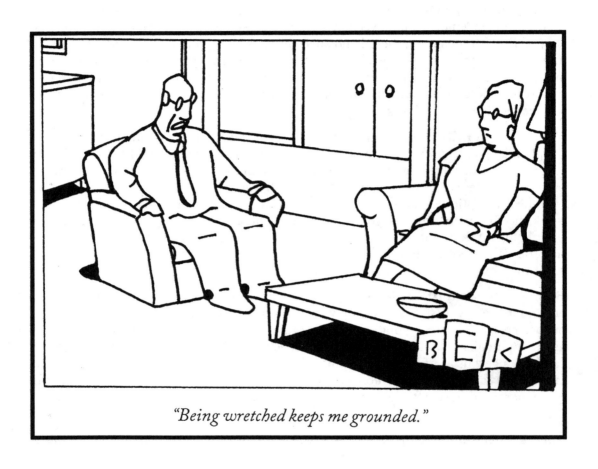

"*Being wretched keeps me grounded.*"

*I hate my boss. He asked, "Why are you two hours late?" I said, "I fell downstairs." He said, "That doesn't take two hours." —**Johnny Carson***

There is zero tolerance for executives with combustible short fuses who attack, freeze, withdraw or storm out. There is even less for spitfires who try to pass the blame. "The buck stops here" is a law not just a slogan. And executives who are long past being productive are no longer tenured. You must plan for the inevitable. Losing thorough-bred horses are sent to stud farms, but you may not be so lucky.

*You can fool too many of the people too much of the time.—**James Thurber***

Teamwork can be dangerous—a category that combines the good, the bad and the ugly.

In unity there is strength: The days of rugged individualism are over. Individuals no longer build great products or full services. They must be members of a team that holds everyone accountable—all the time—and must support each other toward a common goal, with equal responsibilities, aspirations, and encouragement. That's good, but there is one caveat. Friendships don't last forever: peer approval or rejection in business, in social and in athletic endeavors are temporary and can be overturned by new events.

On the other hand, according to author Scott Adams, "A team is often formed with a small number of ineffective personnel who have been reassigned to a place where they can do the least damage." Nothing can be more absurd than putting the least competent people in a boat that requires them to all row in tempo.

*Women in the workplace are overly sensitive. One friend at the employment office was asked if she could make a good cup of coffee. She stormed out of the building before she learned that the employer was Starbucks. —**Carol Leifer***

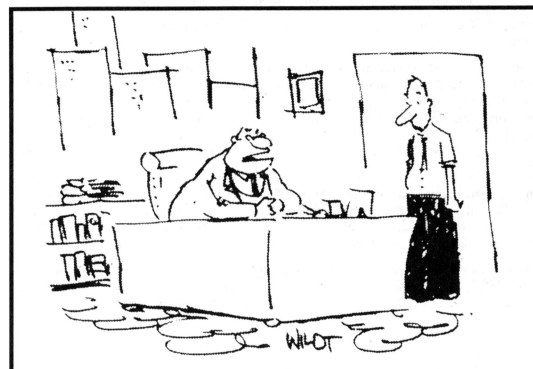

"Well, we used to give our employees the benefit of the doubt. But we're dropping that benefit, too."

Show Me the Money—
Running Your Own Business

*When I was young I thought money was the most important thing in life. And now that I'm old—I know it is.—**Oscar Wilde***

Just for fund: It's called the bottom line because it's the final net figure that always determines whether or not you're equipped to run your own business. Every day is filled with rejections, and there are more than fifty rejection formulas every entrepreneur needs to know. Here are the top formulas on the list that can minimize but never eliminate serious business chaos before it metastasizes.

Sign on street vendor cart: *"I don't want to set the world on fire. I just want to keep my nuts warm."*

Cover your assets: Expect embezzlement and betrayal. Get a financial report every day from your CFO. You may not have time to read it, but only you know that. More businesses have gone belly-up because the owners didn't watch the cash flow that was their business's lifeblood. Suddenly, the bank calls, and you yell "SHIT," which now stands for "shoulda had an intelligent treasurer." Look under the hood of your business more often than you do your car.

Men always scratch their ass when they're thinking, because that's where their brain is.
*—**Tim Allen***

Never fade out: There is a lot of larceny is the world and a little bit in everybody. When you leave money on the table (like giving someone authorization to spend money, sign checks or buy materials), you're foolishly stimulating that instinct. Half the marriages end in divorce, and business partnerships break up more often. And the most common reason is money. Your administrative staff will not only have sticky figures when it comes to dollars, but don't be surprised to find them stealing first your files, then your people, then your reputation, and finally your accounts. The more successful you are, the more you encourage the greedy, not the needy.

*Someday I want to be rich. Some people get so rich they lose all respect for humanity. That's how rich I want to be. —**Rita Rudner***

Starbucks is one long grind: Be on the lookout for any unusual behavior or communication. If you placed your trust in friendship, just remember the Mafia movie line when someone is getting whacked, "It's not personal, it's business."

*I have a lot of friends in very high places. I just hope the police can talk them down. —**Craig Sharf***

Crisis management: Delegate responsibility for work, but not for outcome. You must know every detail of your business. The title of chief operating officer really means you can operate as well as train the personnel in every department. Executives find that they become better managers when they are open to more suggestions. Sir Howard Stringer, CEO of Sony Corporation, claims "I rely upon people who know a lot more than I do. I'm very careful to surround myself with people who fill in a lot of blanks. It has helped me communicate better. I'm open and friendly, and I'm having a good time at work."

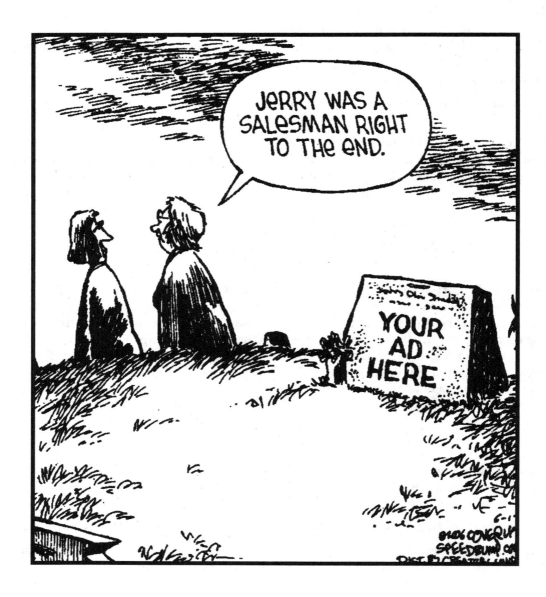

The road to success is always under construction. **—Lily Tomlin**

Abandon a project that is failing. Martha Stewart, who should know better, said in her book *Perfectly Perfect* that "failing is not the problem; not trying is." That is also perfectly stupid advice. When you are too proud to know that the *Titanic* is sinking is when your business will drown. Cut your losses quickly, even if that means firing your best friends and relatives. Working to turn things around is admirable, but hoping that normal business staffing and equipment will eventually correct the problem is an example of amateur night. Focus on projects you not only understand but also can control.

I was one of their most important employees because I ran that company—right into the ground. **—Wendy Liebman**

Hardships prove character. The best employees are smart because they're hungry. Notice that within a year after most major league athletes get their million dollar contracts and endorsement deals, their productivity rapidly declines. It's arguably the most controversial fact in business, but within five years a company will outgrow the initial people who bask in the adoration of having helped start the trail blazing but haven't kept up to the changing paths of the market. The key to success is to get rid of them as painlessly as possible and keep your staff lean and hungry. Remember that the Texas saying, "Dance with the one that brung ya," is only for singing cowboys.

Put the fable on the table: One of the greatest baseball stories is a myth. According to the legend, in 1945, Branch Rickey decided to break the color-line in Major League Baseball by hiring the first black player. He selected Jackie Robinson, but only after he tested Robinson's temper. Rickey questioned him at great length, bellowed out racial epitaphs, and insulted his family, his ability, and his courage. He even pretended to throw a punch at the young man's face. But a forewarned Robinson kept his cool and not only became the first black major leaguer but one of the greatest players of all time. The myth was that Rickey wanted to eliminate color discrimination. As Robinson, a friend of mine, admitted years later, Rickey's sole reason was a desperate need to increase attendance at his Brooklyn Dodgers home games by getting more African-Americans to become fans. "He didn't want a baseball player who didn't have the guts to fight back," said Robinson. "He wanted a ballplayer with guts enough *not* to fight back, so he wouldn't provoke a riot at the ballpark."

Line by line: Your best advertising is word of mouth. People prefer doing business with people they respect. Every person who does business with you—customer or supplier—should be your best salesperson. Once the public trusts your first product, try line extension. Coca-Cola research indicated that the average person drinks 64 ounces of liquid a day. Since the company realized that Coke, by itself, would never be the exclusive fluid, they went into other beverage products like juices (Minute Maid), iced-coffee (Caribou), milk (Swerve), and just plain water (Dasani).

You'll learn to cope with rejection by just fighting and fighting. You'll fail a lot, but then you'll find you're in great company.

Don't hire in your own image: Check your ego at the door. Otherwise, the more successful your business is, the more it controls your life. For example, even though there's no cloud on the horizon, all you can see is a rainbow and the money's green. When

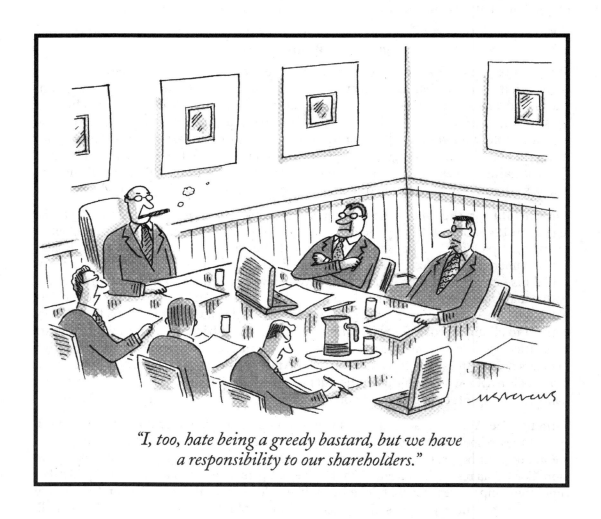

"I, too, hate being a greedy bastard, but we have a responsibility to our shareholders."

you start putting all your eggs in one basket, like not diversifying your customer base, soon one client group has its hands on your business faucet. In the worst-case scenario, you don't react to change quickly enough. You don't have a seatbelt if you have no contingencies in place. And people who said they were on your side are now plunging knifes into your back. They come to bury Caesar, not to praise him.

*People always say, "He died penniless." As if it's a terrible thing. Sounds like good timing, to me. —**Al Cleathen***

Venture capital, the entrepreneur's Achilles' heel: Conventional wisdom claims "Nothing ventured, nothing lost." But it's just not a sound business practice. To grow, you need more and more money for start-up costs and personnel. Ironically, the problems you had when you started the business are compounded now that you're successful. Your needs are geometrically bigger. Banks are of no help, because you kept your account with one bank, instead of two. "It's hard to get big corporations or banks to invest in new big-ticket development products by smaller companies because the risk increases exponentially," predicts Merle Young. So you seek venture capital partners, unaware that venture capital funding can pull the rug from underneath your whole company at any moment. The day the bubble bursts and everyone gets whacked is the day when the massive sucking sound you hear is your company going down the drain.

If lawyers are disbarred and clergymen defrocked, than shouldn't electricians be delighted, musicians denoted, cowboys deranged, models deposed, tree surgeons debarked and dry cleaners depressed?

Focus on sales and service. Traditionally, there are three major ingredients of a successful business—money, product and sales—but one other factor is far more dangerous: letting someone else get between you and your most important customers or clients. Never allow the fate of your business to be in the hands of someone else. When I was learning to ride horses, a wrangler once said to me, "The reason you're on top of the horse is because the horse thinks you're smarter than he is. When the horse finds out he's smarter, he's going to try to get on top." Never let any account person become so vitally important that your customer goes to him first for problem solving. That's why you must personally meet with every VIP client as frequently as possible. All communications—invoices, mail and email—must go to you and through you. All executives must sign non-compete legal contracts that discourage them from jumping ship and pitching your customers. Without them, you are a disaster waiting to happen. Even with them, the signed agreements are more of a threat than a slam-dunk prohibition. Make sure that all agreements are tucked away in your secure file so no one can get his hands on them when the dirt hits the fan. Guerrilla tactics should be a marketing plan, not a personnel option.

The gift of grab: The most common rejection fear in business is not making a profit; it's getting a "no" when trying to make a sale. Yet selling does not even begin until a customer says "no." Until then," says Chris Koch, "you are simply taking an order." Every sale call should end by asking for the order, just as a good speech ends with suggested action. The sales process has four parts: (1) developing a relationship with the customer, (2) identifying the customer's needs, (3) fostering a desire by the customer for your product or service, and (4) making it easy for the customer to say "yes." The last part can be exclusiveness, or a price reduction, or immediate delivery, or money-back satisfaction.

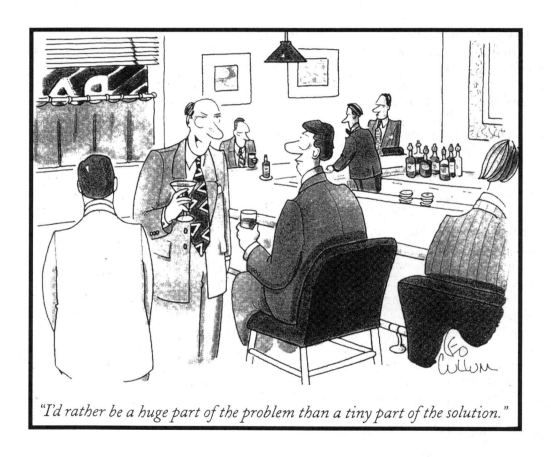

"I'd rather be a huge part of the problem than a tiny part of the solution."

LAP It Up—Getting That Promotion

Odds-on: One of your major rejections may be the failure to get a promotion, salary raise, a step-up position with new responsibilities, or a financial reward. It happens at least once every three to five years. And the odds of victory are four to one against you. The reason for failure may be your sales pitch without adequate preparation. There are three major stages of a well-planned campaign. You just don't walk into a boss's office and demand a raise. Pressuring for a now-or- never fireworks display is likely to detonate a short fuse. Here's the three-stage successful plan.

(1) Love: Break the ice with compliments. Tell your boss (or decision maker) that you love your job, you love your company, and you love him/her. Include statements indicating how happy you have been over the years, how appreciative you are by everyone's encouragement and compliments, and how you support the company's products, objectives, and decisions. By the time you've finished this gushy preamble, your boss should be nodding: "Yes, I am a nice person and yes, they do love me."

(2) Awards: This is the time to turn your "awards" into everyone's "rewards." Your boss wants to know "what's in it for me?" So remember this story:

> *Joseph went to the innkeeper and asked, "Can you give us a room for the night? My wife, Mary, is pregnant." "Why should I," asked the innkeeper, "just because your wife is pregnant? I didn't get any pleasure from that." Joseph looked at him and said, "Neither did I."*

(3) Promotion: Without promotion, said P.T. Barnum, something terrible happens—nothing! Promotion, in the pitch for the raise, makes the future even brighter. Not only will the winning team stay intact, but the raise will be encouragement to redouble your efforts, offer new ideas, and increase company morale. By now, your boss is most likely to say, "Let me see what I can do," And your answer is critical, such as "Wonderful. I'll drop in again tomorrow." "No," says your boss. "I'll need a week." And your answer, to alleviate pressure, is "O.K., no problem." You've successfully put the burden of a quick decision on his shoulders. Unless you're dispensable, he's more likely to approve your request in a few days—not a week.

The above three-stage plan of (1) love, (2) award, and (3) promotion forms an appropriate acronym spelled LAP. It's not only easy to remember, it's an icon for what you're going to have to do anyway.

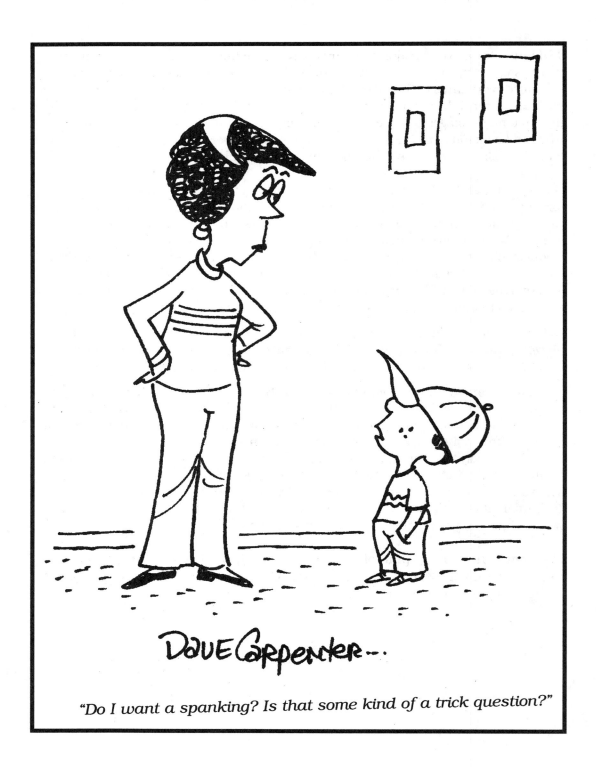

"Do I want a spanking? Is that some kind of a trick question?"

Slam, Bam, Thank You Ma'am—
Studying the Criticism

Two kinds of people fail—those who listen to nobody and those who listen to everybody.

All in the family: Anger and even hatred at stinging criticism is natural, but astute creative people can make the negative a positive. Rejection can burn through most lines of defense. So it's easier if it comes from a professional, but it must be from a professional who has no benefit from your success or failure. That wasn't the case with a young actress, Evan Rachel Wood, who made her professional debut when she was five. Continuing to act in films but attending public school, Wood was harassed by jealous students and even her teachers. "They claimed that I was spoiled and stuck up, so they gave me the hardest time they possibly could." But instead of thinking her rejection came from strangers, she assuaged her feelings by thinking of her critics as a member of her family. She won her classmates over by smiling, joking, and friendly gestures. With siblings, you can disagree, but normally you won't dissolve a relationship or swear yourself into combat.

Talk about criticism. I told my doctor I broke my leg in two places, and he told me to stop going to those places. —Henny Youngman

Don't take a big mistake? Accepting criticism is mandatory when it comes from your boss. The next time your supervisor gives you negative feedback, put your emotions on hold. Consider her objections. Could you have prevented criticism by asking her opinion before you started the assignment? Can you improve your work on the second round by incorporating her ideas? Accepting rejection is not closure. Your work is a continuing activity.

I am always pushed by the negative. The apparent failure of a play sends me back to the typewriter that very night, even before the reviews are in. I'm more compelled to get back to work than if I had a success. —Tennessee Williams

Stay away from my door: Avoid rejection by refusing to get involved with unprofessional critics. According to Carolyn Hax, most unofficial critics aren't worth trying to please, like readers who write book reviews on Amazon.com. "Being polite is fine for the larger world," Hax wrote, "but don't try to counter with your own opinions. Just bite your tongue." Margo Howard adds that back-stabbing tells you that the critic is neither happy nor secure. "The only way such people can feel they're 'in' is to diminish someone else," claims Howard.

Enemy in cite: On the other hand, the best way to respond to authorized criticism is to consider your critic to be a worthy opponent in a game in which you want to become proficient. The better your opponent, the better you play. As Joshua Halberstam wrote in *Everyday Ethics,* "make your enemy work for you, not eat away at you."

Don't Let the Bastards Get You Down

Now Hear This—Getting a Second Opinion

On my last visit, my doctor asked me, "What's wrong? I told him that I couldn't pee. He asked, "How old are you?" I said, "About 80." He said, "You've peed enough." I said, "I want a second opinion," and he said, "O.K., come back tomorrow."

Even a broken clock is accurate twice a day: After one month, it can boast of a series of 60 successes. Don't be overconfident. Too much pride from yesterday's accomplishments is not dependable as a forecaster of tomorrow. Seek second opinions from the most experienced advisors you can find, yet expect that there are always going to be new factors that can wash out tomorrow's victory parade. Don't expect miracles. The race may be won by the beautiful and the just, but that's not the way to bet.

The NFL cheerleaders are gorgeous, but are their cheers helping anybody? Ever see a player interviewed after the game who said, "We were down pretty big in the fourth quarter, but then the cheerleaders started shouting "Defense! Defense!" That's when it dawned on the coach, "Them gals are right." —Gary Culman

The wizard of ahhs. According to Carol Frank, in her book *Do as I Say, Not as I Did!* "Outsiders believe in myths. They don't know much about your business from the outside and they expect positive results all the time and are quick to criticize."

If you think nobody cares if you're alive, try missing a couple of car payments.

A bell-ringer: A couple in Massachusetts were incensed that they were not invited to a friend's wedding, although they did give expensive gifts when they attended the preliminary engagement party and bridal shower. The excuse from the family was that they needed to cut expenses and only immediate relatives were invited. So the disappointed couple asked the opinion of Carolyn Hax of the *Washington Post,* who counseled that "they should accept the fact—from decent people doing their best under highly charged circumstances—that it's not personal, it's just business. In these cases," said Hax, "it is best not to show your lack of maturity of social graces and just keep your mouth shut."

The loan arranger: When David Banks got laid off driving an 18-wheel semi, he decided to go into the detailing business on his own. He needed to buy equipment to clean and wax car exteriors, shampoo carpets, and clean the engine compartment. But no bank in Columbia, Arkansas, would arrange a loan because he had a spotty credit rating and no previous business experience. But he got a second opinion from his lawyer. Do your own banking. He went to used car dealers in town, who wanted their cars spotless before being put on the lot, offered a rate lower than competitors with guaranteed no-pay satisfaction, and got enough advance contracts to get started. Within a year, he was expanding to two other Arkansas cities.

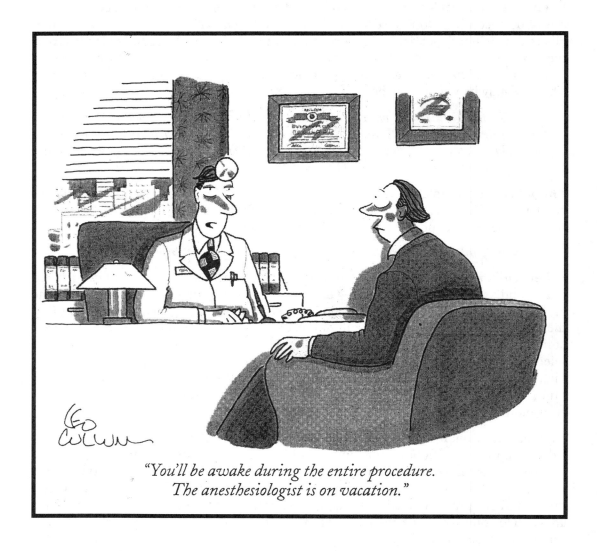

"You'll be awake during the entire procedure.
The anesthesiologist is on vacation."

One Damp Thing After Another— Testing the Waters

*Millions long for immortality, yet they still don't know what to do with themselves on a rainy Sunday afternoon. —**Susan Ertz***

Test the water: Before plunging into any endeavor, serious research, sometimes called a feasibility study, is strongly recommended. This involves not only library research, but also a lot of interviewing of target individuals. For example, researching present and past employees of a firm interviewing you for a job makes sense. Just as you check *Consumer's Digest* before buying a refrigerator, it also makes sense to find out as much as you can about a boss that will be a major part of your life for some time to come.

*I'm not superstitious. It just brings bad luck. —**Placido Domingo***

Penny wise: To quickly check the life of your car's tires, place a penny in the tire's treads with the top of Lincoln's head pointing down. If you can see the top of Lincoln's head, the tire is worn and needs replacing. Similarly there are obvious tests to check the financial aspects of any decision. It may sound crass to some altruists, but if something is not worth doing for money, it's probably not worth doing at all.

*You never get into trouble for the things you didn't say. —**Sam Rayburn***

Yes, sir! Running a business as a boss is not unlike being a general in a battle. Driven rulers have little time for a democratic vote on every offense. Executive decision makers, often portrayed in films as tyrannical (think Gordon Gekko, the Wall Street corporate raider, as portrayed by Michael Douglas, or Miranda Priestly, the high fashion priestess, as portrayed by Meryl Streep), demand support as well as awe. Most of their decisions are arbitrary and self-serving. But if you're going to pocket their weekly salary, you've got to agree to stomach their humiliations.

Arguing with reality is like trying to teach a cat to bark—hopeless.

Help me: Bosses are eager for a plan to succeed. So, while hatching an innovative project, it might be wise to show your supervisor a preliminary version. If it succeeds, she'll certainly share the credit for it, but if it fails she'll certainly finger you for the blame. But Monica Ramirez Basco, in her book *Never Good Enough,* claims it's easier to accept criticism before you've polished a project, and factoring in a soft deadline will help you get started earlier.

*The best way to give advice to other people is to find out what they want and then advise them to do it. —**Harry S. Truman***

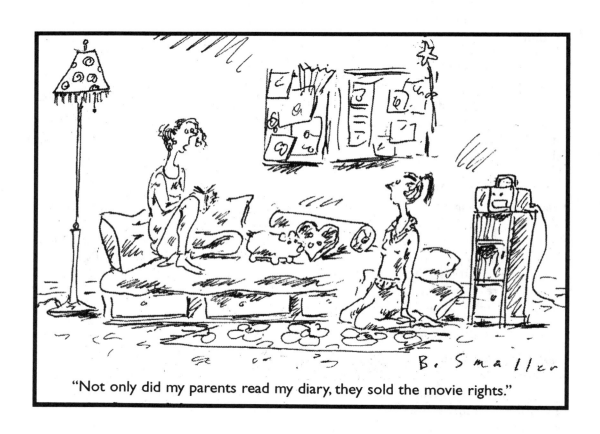

"Not only did my parents read my diary, they sold the movie rights."

A Private Affair—
Minding Your Own Business

You can avoid most controversies by minding your own business. Like the best way to avoid a shark attack is to stay the hell out of the water. It's their territory.

Ignorance is bliss: You're looking for trouble when you read papers or mail on your neighbor's desk or mailbox. When people have inadvertently left confidential information, like divorce papers or even a resume, on the copying machine, resist the temptation to read it in detail and add to the local gossip. According to Jared Sandberg of *The Wall Street Journal,* "There seems to come a time when many people would prefer to remain out of the loop." He claims that while gossip has its appeal, having too much disparaging information about someone else can not only show disrespect, it can reflect badly on you. "Your life is happier," wrote Sandberg, "when you don't know all the dirty little secrets that go on with your friends."

It is a sin to believe evil of others, but it is seldom a mistake. —*H.L. Mencken*

Out of the closet: Time and time again, celebrities—in entertainment or the government—find that trying to cover up a negative story only gets them in deeper water. The best solution is to make a public announcement and then disappear even if the gossip doesn't. It will eventually because something new happens tomorrow. When Cynthia Nixon was one of the stars in TV's *Sex and the City,* she met and fell in love with another woman and broke up with the father of her two children. She tried to keep the affair a secret, but the media and prying paparazzi kept hounding her. Rather than hide, Nixon simply acknowledged the relationship and refused to say anything further. Within a few weeks, the furor petered out. "When someone is chasing you," she said. "Stop running. And they'll stop, too."

Don't go public: Don't take one slight or rejection and enlarge its significance by a letter to an editor or a lawsuit. Even with a defamatory news article, only a small percentage of the public will have read it. So when you turn a minor cause celebre into a firebomb, people want to know "what was all the fuss about?" and the repeated defamation gets more widely circulated.

Face your own shortcomings: As a teenager Jonathan Franzen was a nerd. Then, a few years later, he wrote a best selling book, *The Corrections,* and publicly insulted Oprah Winfrey's invitation to be on her show. "I had received so much attention—good and bad," he said, "that I had a burning feeling of being unrecognized for what I felt myself to be. So I made a list of things that were least suitable for public consumption and I decided to write about them to try to forgive myself for making myself a laughable figure." His new book *The Discomfort Zone* is largely the story of how Franzen shed his fears, or at least learned to live with them.

ZIGGY

TOM WILSON

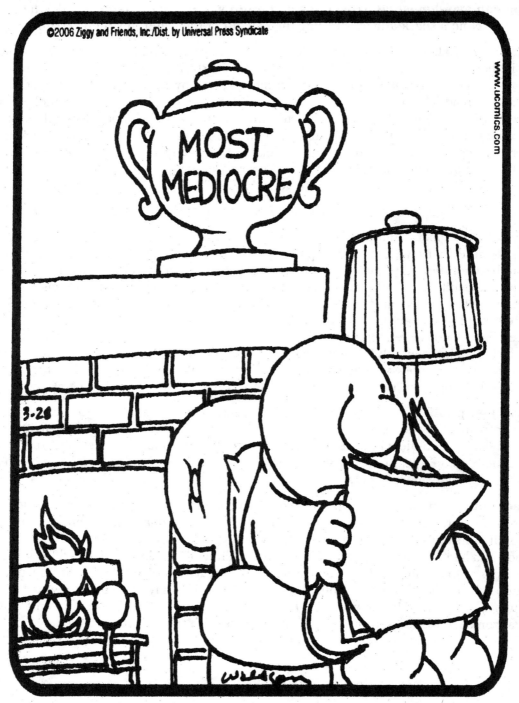

Ordinary People—Lowering Your Expectations

*A girl phoned me the other night and said, "Come on over. Nobody's home." So I rushed over, and she was right. Nobody was home. —**Rodney Dangerfield***

Take it down a notch: The "lower your expectations" theory is one of the most controversial strategies for avoiding rejection. If you don't expect to win the game, make the sale, have a manuscript accepted, be cast for a major theatrical part, or get a date on Saturday night, you've decreased the major stimulant for rejection. Since you know that the odds are against you, just lower your expectations. Others point out that accepting the logical inevitability of rejection permits an enthusiastic posture when you wish to change a negative into a positive. You'll be more appreciative when you do win once in a while, and less depressed when you lose.

I say to kids, you tried your best and you failed miserably. The lesson is, never try. If you don't want the dentist to hurt you, keep your mouth shut.

Balance: You can destroy yourself by striving for perfection, which, obviously, is impossible. "If the focus is perpetual perfection, there is no peace," claims Alexandra Stoddard in *The Art of the Possible*. "The way to have some perfect moments is to free yourself from guilt, from compulsions, from frustrations and unnecessary anguish." Perfection not only causes anxiety, it is the enigma of a person in crisis. There is no room for spontaneity or pleasure. Sogyal Rinpoche, in *The Tibetan Book of Living and Dying*, explained, "Our task is to strike a balance, to find a middle way, to learn not to overstretch ourselves with extraneous activities."

Artists who seek perfection in everything can not attain it in anything.
*—**Eugene Delacroix***

On the other hand: Counter arguments, like those in the best-selling book *The Secret*, are that you should always expect to win the game (or why play?) and that you should go into every encounter filled with the confidence of victory. The claim is you should visualize yourself getting the trophy at the victory dinner, making the Academy Award acceptance speech, cashing the winning lottery ticket, and making love to a future trophy spouse.

*I have a girlfriend that is beautiful, sexy, intelligent and very passionate. I think she's wonderful. But, my wife, on the other hand . . . pfff! —**Jackie Mason***

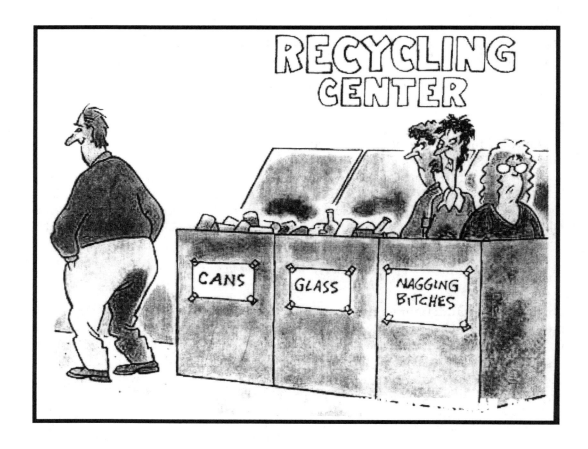

Pay as You Glow—
Buying Your Way Out of Trouble

Every man is a damn fool for at least five minutes a day. Wisdom consists of not exceeding the limits. **—Elbert Hubbard**

Pay the two dollars: There's an old vaudeville sketch about a man who tries to get out of the two-dollar parking ticket by compounding his problem with a wide variety of scheming, denial, and bombastic threats. Before he's done, the fines have been upgraded so that he ends up going to the gallows. There are times when you must cut your losses and accept defeat graciously. If your ego becomes too rigid, you can crack. As a result, many well-to-do people, especially celebrities in sports and entertainment, will pay off their accusers immediately rather than fight them publicly in the media or the courts. The lesson is that often surrender is the wisest course of valor.

When her husband died, his wife put the usual death notice in the paper, but added he died of gonorrhea. The next day, a family friend phoned and said, "Sara, you know very well he died of diarrhea, not gonorrhea." The elderly widow said, "I nursed him day and night for over 50 years, so of course I know he died of diarrhea. I just thought it would be better for posterity to remember him as a great lover than a big piece of crap."

Charity begins in prison: In 1987, Michael Milken was the most dynamic and highly paid person in American finance. Perhaps too dynamic! Three years later he pleaded guilty to six felonies, including conspiracy, fraud, the filing of false security information, and market manipulation. The SEC estimated that his crimes had cost investors more than a billion dollars. He was convicted, fined a billion dollars, and sent to prison. To win probation, he agreed to devote himself to charitable endeavors.

Pardon me: He founded the Milken Family Foundation, which awarded $40 million to 1,600 teachers and administrators in awards that averaged $25 thousand each. He also established a college scholarship program for needy students. He embraced an array of mental, physical, and spiritual techniques, from meditation to holistic diets, plus donated millions of dollars to organizations for prostate-cancer research. While he claimed all this was an attempt to "give back and make us better at what we are doing," skeptics were convinced it was mainly being done as public relations efforts to persuade the President to issue him a pardon.

Some habits are hard to break: But just as criminals often go back to the scene of their crime, Milken could not live up to one promise he made to the S.E.C., and that was to be barred for life from any association as an investment advisor, broker, or securities dealer. By the time the government's second investigation of his activities was completed, Milken was forced to pay an additional $47 million as a "disgorgement fee plus interest," and President Clinton left office without issuing Milken the pardon he felt he had bought but not earned.

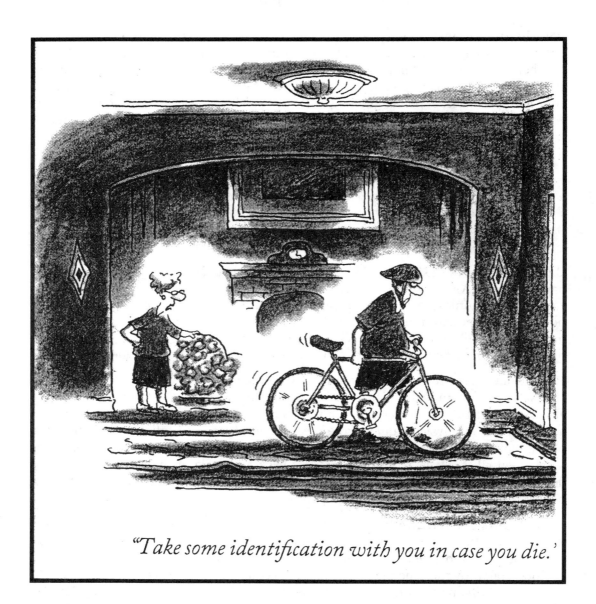

"Take some identification with you in case you die.'

Shoot the Messenger—Protecting Your Ass

Life isn't like a box of chocolates. It's like a jar of jalapenos. You never know what's going to burn your ass. —**Paul Rodriguez**

The gang's all here: Forging alliances by getting, in advance, the support of your peers is essential, claims Dr. Laurie Anderson. Your chances of being blindsided will be far less if you have the prior endorsement of your colleagues. Leaders need each other. They think in terms of "we" rather than "I." Each party must believe there will not be a success without the other.

Even with the best of schemes, nothing offers 100% protection. Like condoms. A friend of mine was wearing one and got hit by a bus. —**Bob Rubin**

Protect your ass: There's no reason to be salacious, but making sure your reputation goes unharmed is a necessity. "A memorandum," said Dean Acheson, "is written not to inform the reader but to protect the writer." According to Jared Sandberg of *The Wall Street Journal,* it's called corporate dodgeball, during which executives begin a close, lifetime relationship with their file folders. Self-protection is a full-time job in any public or private organization. According to Jerry Flynn, a VP of human resources, "It's become a way of life to document conversations and written missives, as well as copies of contracts and orders." While it's unpleasant to expect the worse, deadlines can trigger unplanned outcomes that are emotionally fueled. Failure to document your legal actions is an expensive way to learn. "I really hate living this way," Flynn admits, "but all it takes is being burned once or twice."

Trust your husband, adore your husband, and get as much in your own name as you can. —**Joan Rivers**

Why is it that we never have time to do it right, but we can find time to do it over? We live in a performance based culture. Corporate teams are coached to build relationships that can achieve break-through performance improvements. And members of the team are judged on what they did, not on what they promised. That's why it's important to communicate performance standards so all members of the team have accurate information to help them do their jobs, which start today not tomorrow. "As an example, if you like to debate," says author Tom Peters, "you attract fellow debaters. On the other hand, if you go out on a limb to chase your dreams, you'll attract leaders."

It's results that count and formal performance reviews do nothing to help job performances, according to Jim Trinka. Leadership no longer focuses on correcting weaknesses but on focusing on each employee's profound strengths. Research indicates this method produces as much as 80 percent increase in break-through performance activity.

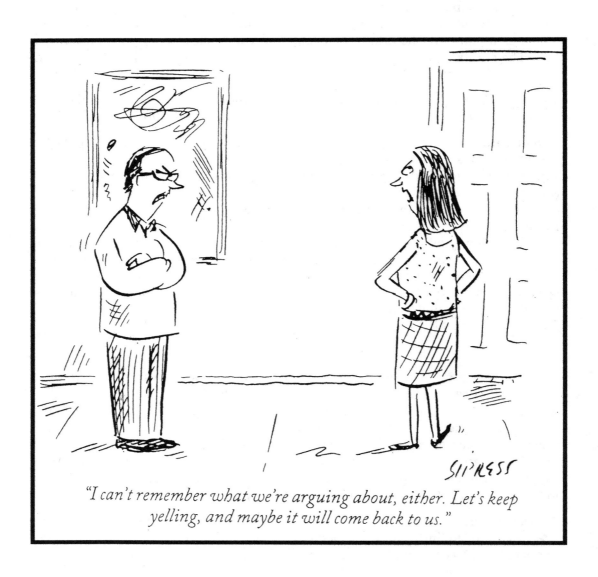

"I can't remember what we're arguing about, either. Let's keep yelling, and maybe it will come back to us."

Conversation Peace—
Negotiate and Compromise

When my wife and I argue, she wins only 50 percent of the time. The other 50 percent of the time, my mother-in-law wins.

Everyone wins: We complicate matters when we assume that there are opposing sides. The challenge is to find the issues that promote a common goal so that both parties can agree on something tangible. Patricia Wheeler lists five keys that can turn difficult interactions into solution-oriented conversations: (1) put yourself in the other person's shoes—or at least his underwear, (2) acknowledge your desire for improvement, not victory, (3) make requests for change, not demands, (4) compliment the other party for helping create a cordial relationship, and (5) recommend a time to revisit unresolved issues and propose a compromise that makes it easy for your adversary to accept. For example, in a restaurant, when the food is unacceptable, suggest a different menu selection rather than hope you'll get the entire check cancelled. If a hotel room is unacceptable, suggest a different room and then ask for a free dinner. Rather than a "take it or leave it" approach, offer options that are acceptable to you and then leave the choice up to the other side.

Half-baked: Remember that "splitting the difference" is not necessarily fair. One side may have demanded 125 percent of the settlement, so when they offer to split, they end up getting 62.5 percent rather than 50 percent.

Whenever I let my conscience be my guide, I get picked up for vagrancy. —Bob Thaves

Be persistent: "Press on," said McDonald's founder Ray Kroc. "Nothing in the world can take the place of persistency and determination." This admonition works as well for governments as it does for people. When voters reject school or building levies, local governments are entitled to use public funds to put those levies on the ballot again and again until voters finally approve.

Only those who risk going too far can possibly find out how far they can go. —T.S. Eliot

According to Michelangelo, "The great tragedy of life is not that people set their sights too high and fail to achieve their goals, but they set their sights too low and do." Michelangelo was wrong. Just because something doesn't happen the way you planned doesn't mean it's useless. You may find the less successful result was quite satisfactory. What makes you believe that your original expectations were accurate?

The administration insists that one of the best ways to help our balance of trade is to encourage our kids to go south of the border to buy drugs and send our senior citizens north of the border to buy drugs. —Mel Helitzer

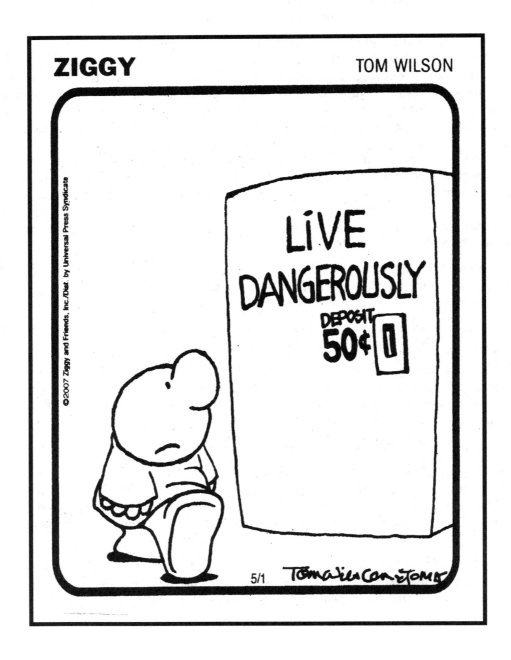

Cool It—59 Catalysts for Positive Action

Even though you can't go back and make a new start, you can start now and make a new ending.

The heart of most rejections is human choice. So you must consider the judge as well as the judgment. If you've been left out, yet have respect for the source, you may discover a flaw that needs correction. If you're not defective merchandise, you're still saleable.

Is rejection of you an act to compensate for their own aggressive humiliation? Or is it an attempt to damage your reputation or an effort by someone to advance himself?

Rejection can be a wake-up call, claims psychologist John Preston. "What if I had only six months to live," he questioned. "Would I be as depressed as I am right now?" Sometimes that can put things in perspective, but it should not stop there. It should ignite some kind of action.

A frequent rebuttal against literary critics is they might have been rejected in their own artistic submissions and thus are getting even by unloading against you! A better rebuttal is to hope public opinion overwhelms the professional critics. When Glenna Goodacre sculpted her Vietnam Women's Memorial in Washington, two major critics, including Maya Lin, creator of the famous Vietnam Veterans Memorial, snubbed her statues as kitsch. However, she was able to get over the poor reviews when large groups of women, who were the focus of the memorial, wrote about how the sculpture helped them deal with the war and how it had changed their lives. "I found which was more important," said Goodacre. "A positive response from those women or a good review from some critic."

Some people (or publications) thrive on gossip as self-appointed gatekeepers of information that others want to be the first to know. Both groups are harmful. "Hearing about the shortcomings of others, true or not, somehow makes some people feel more secure in their existence," says Hap LeCrone, a Cox News columnist. Some friends are pessimistic of your plans or endeavors by their own insecurity. If they can't do it, they believe neither can you.

If you are skeptical of any critic, write down your misgivings. Develop a "What's the worst that can happen?" list. This will give you a chance to think about it, but be open; rejection is not all negative or unworthy. Even the most devious of opponents may point to some kernel of truth.

The following list of rejection remedies are not ranked by any numerical or approval rating. Perhaps only one or two are best suited for each individual circumstance, and many are so extreme that they are not advisable for everyone. But once you find the solutions that work for you, stay with them. Don't mess with success.

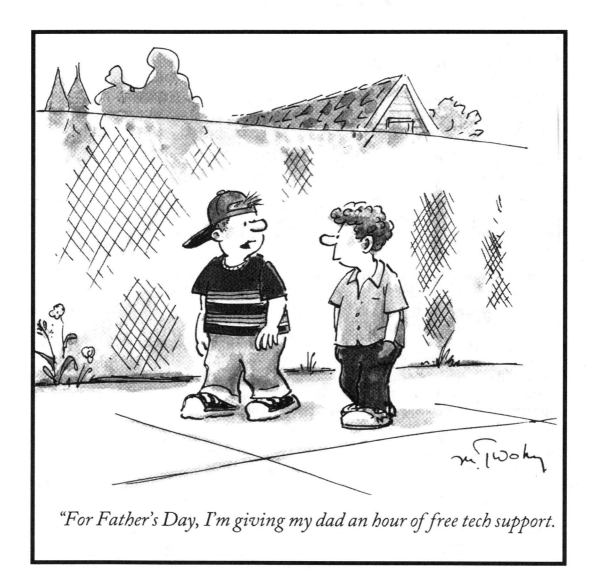

"For Father's Day, I'm giving my dad an hour of free tech support.

The Slime Machine—The Computer Rules

According to a survey, 85 percent of men admit they surf the Internet wearing only their underwear. 63 percent said that's how they lost their last job. —Jay Leno

Yes, icon: Our heart may be ruled by God, but our minds are ruled by technology. Today, the most popular escape from rejection is the time- and mind-absorbing immersion required by computer games and online gambling.

My heart belongs to data: The first computer games, the genesis of today's biggest new industry, were serious designs by RAND (acronym for Research and Development) intellectuals in the early days of the Cold War on how to plan for the apocalypse of nuclear war—how to prevent it, how to win it or how to survive Doomsday. They were eggheads in a world of meatheads, and their mandarin was Herman Kahn, who not only had the highest I.Q. on record but also claimed he could only postulate such a grotesque fantasy of massive retaliation with high speed computer science and mind-boggling systems analysis.

The real reason Abraham Lincoln was shot in the theater was because his cell phone kept going off. —Jay Leno

Bang, bang. You're dead: Half a century later, anyone with a computer and internet access can play war games, and while they have yet to equal the preposterous realism of thermonuclear wars, each week sees the marketing of games with complex bells and whistles that have a quality equal to high density TV. Since *Pong* was introduced in the 1970's, computer geeks can also play sports, cops and robbers, and take target practice against earthly terrorists or space invaders. A video football game, *Madden NFL,* sold more than $100 million in one week, equaling the seven-day gross of *The Da Vinci Code,* one of Hollywood's highest-grossing films. The fastest segment of the game market is people over 40 who are willing to be rewired to learn new skills.

Hard drive is not a sexual act: But the biggest escape in Internet town is on-line gambling. Off-track betting on thoroughbred racing and all major sports has been around for decades, but today you can also play blackjack, the nation's favorite casino game, plus slots, craps, roulette, and a dozen other break-your-chops games without leaving home. In fact, more people are participating in Internet poker games than all the people combined playing poker at casinos around the world. So many billions of dollars are being bet on-line that no one can accurately estimate the take, because Internet gambling is unregulated, unlimited and illegal in the U.S. The habit has overwhelmed the I.R.S., which is losing billions in uncollectable tax revenue. And educators are forced to admit that the popularity of on-line games is the biggest anchor drowning students of all ages from required reading, writing, and interpersonal communication.

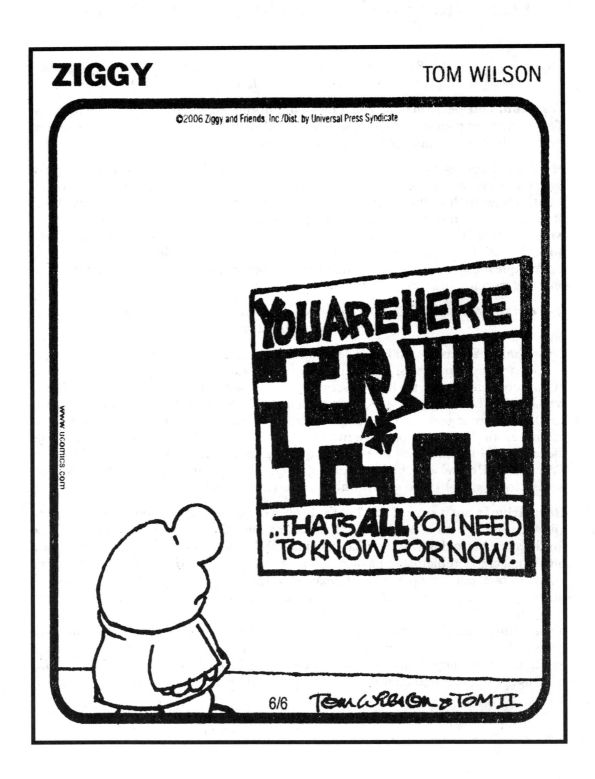

Time's Up—Relax and Take It Easy

It's never too late to do nothing at all. —***Allen Ginsberg***

Doing nothing is doing something: When they're preparing you for takeoff, stewardesses always urge you to fasten your seat belt and then "sit back and relax." It's good rejection action advice, too. Some, like Samuel Johnson, claim that "all intellectual improvement arises from leisure." We doubt this is true. We would put our money on necessity as a more stimulating motivator.

The (Lewinsky) affair was a wacko deal for the nation, but it turned out to be kind of liberating for me. It's easier to beat your demons if you let them go, and I have.
—***Bill Clinton***

It's natural to feel unhappy: Just as predictably, 90% of all rejections can be ameliorated by relaxation and unemotional behavior. That's natural, too. Take a shower, a Jacuzzi or a spell in the hot tub. Downside, this may be a short-term solution, but it does have the upside of giving you time for your mind to cool off while your body absorbs the heat. Rodgers and Hammerstein wrote in their musical *South Pacific,* "I'm Gonna Wash That Man Right Out of My Hair," a song that proved popular not only because of its tune but also because of its widespread acceptance as a rejection tonic.

People are just about as happy as they make up their minds to be. —***Abraham Lincoln***

Fast food: The problem for most of us is that Americans just don't take enough time to relax. Lunch hours are averaging 31 minutes, and the traditional two-week vacation is used by only 14 percent of the working class. Like the old farmer joke that every time he took a day off, when he got back to the farm he found himself two days behind, we often find that we have to hustle to get ahead of our workload in order to leave with our responsibilities under control, and then we have to work overtime when we return just to catch up with our workload. According to Po Bronson, "Today, grownups turn vacations into such active leisure that we exhaust ourselves trying to relax."

Dr. Phil proclaimed the way to achieve inner peace is to finish all the things you've started. So yesterday I looked around and found a lot of things I never finished, like a bottle of Baileys, a half bottle of Grey Goose, a package of Oreos, the remainder of Prozac and Valium, two pieces of cheesecake, a box of pretzels and five pieces of chocolate. You have no idea how freaking good I feel today.

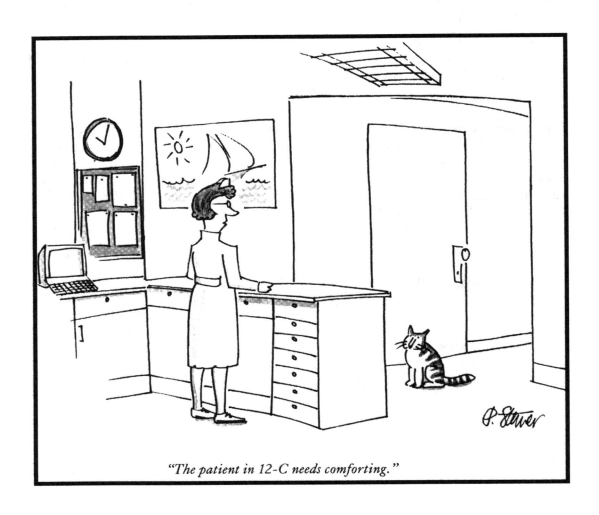

"*The patient in 12-C needs comforting.*"

How to Enjoy a Licking—Adopting a Pet

They say a dog is man's best friend, but I don't buy it. How many times have you had your friends neutered? —**Larry Reeb**

A room with a zoo: When you need comfort, some men even prefer dogs to wives. The dogs understand who's master, they'll listen patiently to all complaints, eat out of your hand—after all, dogs know bitches—and they already have a fur coat. Not to be outdone, many women claim pets are more preferable than men. They are more trustworthy, they protect you, and they can lick their own balls.

Zsa Zsa Gabor, holding her favorite cat, asked Johnny Carson on his Tonight Show if he would like to pet her pussy. "Sure," said Carson, "but first you'll have to move the cat."

Go to the dogs: That's why pets stand out in a forest of pals when you need your body licked. To get prepared for his new job as president of a major corporation, a new CEO put salt on his ass and went to a petting zoo.

My husband and I are either going to buy a dog or have a child. We can't decide whether to ruin our carpet or ruin our lives. —**Rita Rudner**

Lap dogs: There is a recent category of dogs trained as animal-assisted therapy teams to help ailing patients recover lost motor skills or even relearn how to smile. Their calm confidence is contagious. So, too, is their willingness to get into bed with you, be petted and hugged, and even return the favor with sloppy kisses of their own.

I have a dog, and I trained him to go on the paper, but I get so mad when he won't wait until I've finished reading it. —**Richard Jeni**

Seeing-eye dogs: Besides unqualified friendship, pets are beneficial to your health, as long as you don't nuzzle them immediately after they've used the toilet as a drinking fountain. Young puppies will force you to get outside and exercise. You can't send them out into the world without supervision. And for you, as well as the dog, the fresh air is always invigorating, and cold air hitting your face and upper body melts tension and stress.

I told a friend I bought a new dog for $1,500. It was part Airedale and part bull. "What part is bull?" asked the friend. "The part about the $1,500."

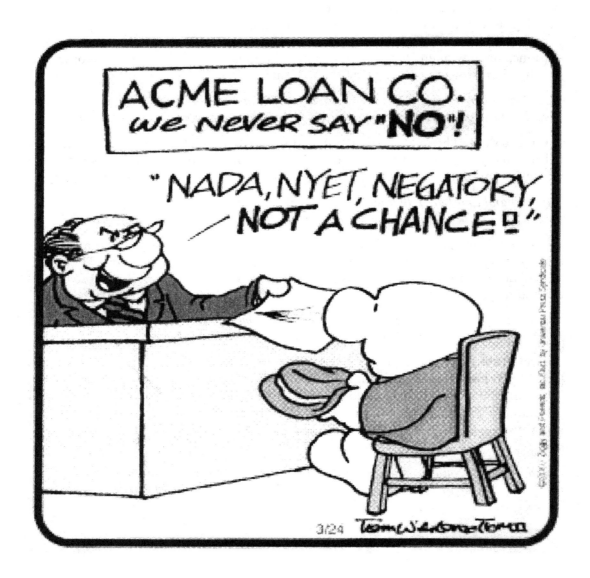

Ja Hable French—Learning a New Language

There was a lot of excitement last week when President Bush was caught on a live microphone pronouncing a four-letter word. What would have been more exciting would be if they caught him pronouncing a four-syllable word. It should be a requirement that the President of the United States be fluent in at least one language. —**Buck Henry**

The war of words: The days of the ugly American are over, when we insisted that foreign guests or trading partners speak English. One world does not mean one language, and when you are dejected, learning a new language can have multiple benefits.

The reason French is so hard to learn is that they have a word for everything.
—Steve Martin

Olé: Spanish has become this country's second language, and if you work in southern states, from Florida to California, that language is so essential that consideration was even given to permitting our National Anthem to be sung in Spanish. "I always thought it was," said one comic. "After all, aren't the first few words 'José, can you see?'"

I bought one of those tapes that teach you to speak Spanish in your sleep. During the night, the tapes kept slipping. Now I speak Spanish with a constant stutter.
—Steven Wright

It's all Greek to me: Midwest students, unfortunately, are not yet living in the 21st century when it comes to international communication. The fault may lie with high schools still teaching Italian, Latin, French, German, and Greek as required languages. Today, college students who study Spanish, as well as Japanese, Chinese, and Russian, are able to hit the ground running when it comes to employment in business, international relations, and media communication. And the Mideast conflict forced Americans, ignorant of the various dialects of Arabic, to act like the blind walking through a minefield.

Take my word for it: Josef Ackerman, CEO of a major bank, vents his rejection anger by studying a new language. Since he already knows four languages fluently, it's likely he has deterred a lot of remorse. He takes his wife on a four-week trip to the country of his new language so the two of them can encourage each other. His theory is total immersion: four weeks with one teacher, and hours each day talking to residents in shops, restaurants, and entertainment venues. "You are able to forge strong connections when you demonstrate you've made the effort to learn someone's native language," he said.

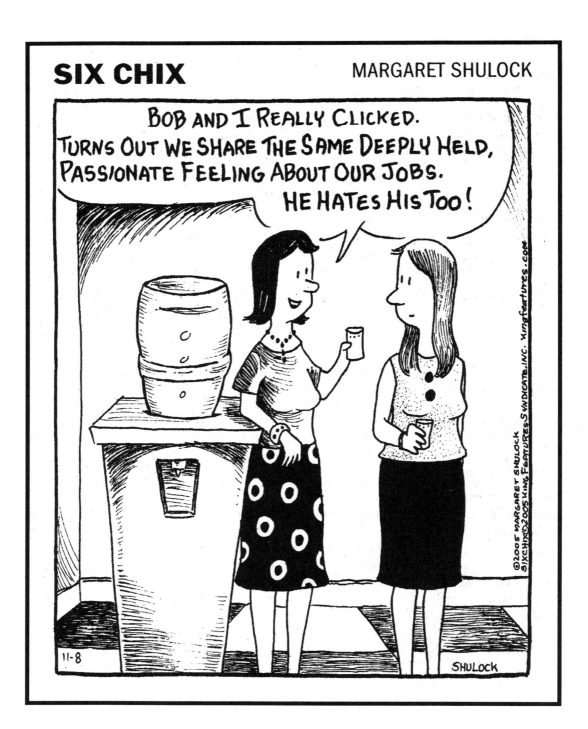

Take This Job and Love It—Acting Your Wage

Pleasure in the job puts perfection in the work. —***Aristotle***

See all the colors of the rainbow: The best thing about being able to think of the future is that it always starts tomorrow. Hillary Clinton's book *It Takes a Village* was a best seller for many reasons, not the least of which was the value of a greater community and the need for interconnecting in order to survive. Reaching out particularly makes sense during the initial healing of a rejection. Every community has a growing list of volunteer outreach organizations. Donating financially is beneficial to the community, but often not to yourself. On the other hand, active participation is a double-barreled benefit. By helping others you end up helping yourself.

Who you are inside is eventually what you look like outside.

The prodigy: By the time she was 13, Michelle Wie became the youngest person—male or female—to win a national adult U.S. Golf Association championship. She was also six feet tall and beautiful. The media heralded her as a child prodigy whose international celebrity would eclipse Tiger Woods. In one year she became the highest paid woman athlete in the world from prize money and endorsements that exceeded $20 million annually. Then, her world suddenly turned flat and contradictory. Trying to compete against male pros, she was cut after the second round in ten tournaments. She was the subject of untold jealousy as sexist criticism suggested that she stay in her own women's tour, and predictions flew that she would shortly flame out. The public apprehension was nixed by Michelle's continuous feisty spirit and her ability to shrug off criticism. "I just refuse to let other people's opinions ruin my life. If people don't like my attitude, they can raise their own daughters to do the things the way they want." Then she added "Oh, wow!" because she is still a teen-ager.

I know a man who gave up smoking, drinking, sex, and rich food. He was healthy right up to the day he killed himself. —***Johnny Carson***

Seven blocks of grant-it: You don't have to love your job to do it well. The secret is being organized. Here are seven tips by Maria Garcia, author of *Get Organized Now:* (1) set goals, (2) make lists, don't rely on your memory, (3) keep a calendar in front of you, (4) group small activities for one period of the day, (5) prepare Q & A in advance of important telephone calls you will make, (6) set early, false deadlines for yourself, and (7) keep papers in clear file folders.

There is no such thing as a self-made man. He is the sum of hard work and all the people who ran to help him as soon as they found out he could do things for himself.
—***Mel Helitzer***

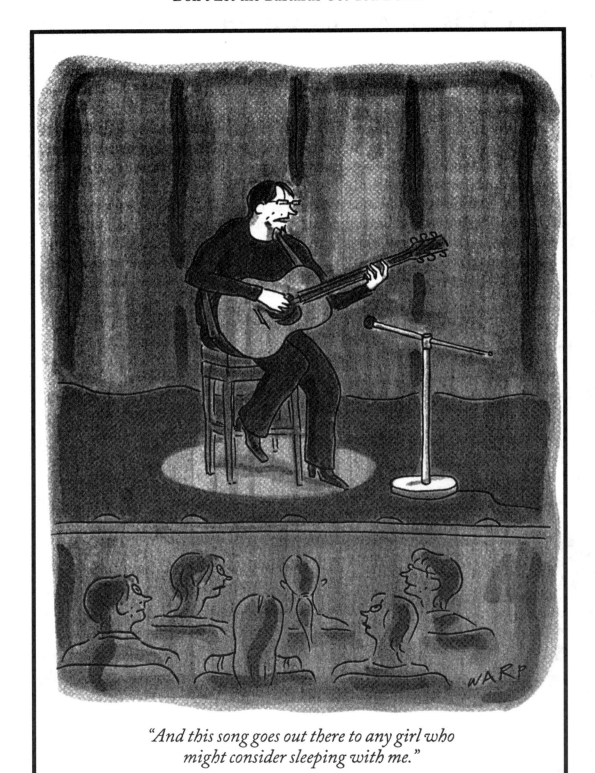

"And this song goes out there to any girl who might consider sleeping with me."

I'm Singing in My Brain—Music as Therapy

*I never get the blues. I sing 'em. —**Eric Burdon***

Just whistle a happy tune: A written message of hope can be read once or twice, but a song can be sung (or hummed) over and over. A high percentage of songs use rejection as their theme because the theme has such a powerful emotional tug. Rejection is the theme of the lyrics of Negro spirituals like "Nobody Knows the Trouble I've Seen," to Broadway show tunes like "Alone," "Let's Call the Whole Thing Off," and "Smile."

I get a bang out of you: The benefit of music therapy will reinforce your rock 'n soul. Currently, folk and country and western music have the highest percentage of rejection themes with such unsophisticated titles about misfortune, such as *"Baby, don't leave me,"* or *"Baby, why did you leave me?"* or *"We were about to be wed, but I shot her instead—why wait?"* Pete Seeger, who did more to make people aware of the therapy of folk music than any other performer, often said, "A folk singer is only a tool for a song that people sing to themselves to console themselves for losses and hardship."

*I don't like country music. But I don't like to denigrate those who do. And for those people who like country music, denigrate means to "put down." —**Bob Newhart***

Battle of the network stars: Most major celebrities in entertainment, politics, and sports contribute large sums to their favorite charities. But neophyte stars, whose popularity is just bubbling, contribute to quality causes by combining their talent. An example is Greg Grunberg, star of TV's *Heroes,* whose 7-year-old son was diagnosed with epilepsy. Grunberg formed a musical group of fellow celebrities, called "The Battle of the Network Stars," that raised thousands of dollars per concert. "Suddenly, in unity, we had a personal connection to a worthwhile cause," said Grunberg.

Music on a high note: For more than 25 years, Beverly Sills was America's most celebrated native-born opera and concert soprano. But as soon as she stepped off-stage, she immediately transformed into her biggest role, that of a mother of two handicapped children. One was a daughter who was deaf, and the other was a son who was mentally challenged. "The opinion of music critics had lost their meaning," said Sills. "I learned to sing to please myself." People who saw her only in public called her consistently happy. "But I wasn't happy," she admitted. "I was cheerful. The difference is that a person who's happy has no problems. A person who is cheerful has learned to overcome them."

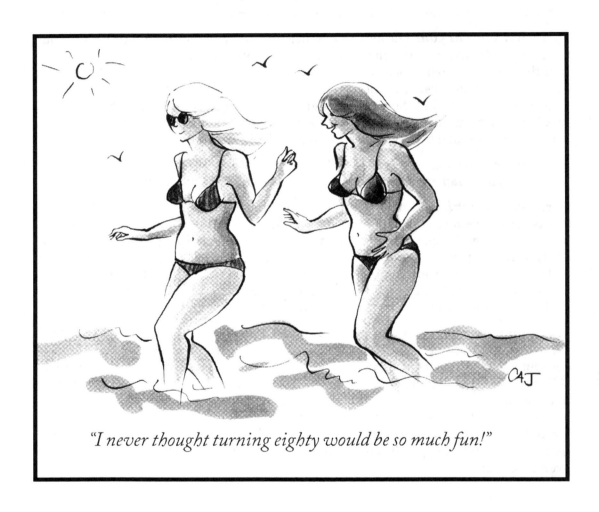

"I never thought turning eighty would be so much fun!"

Swing and Sway Your Cares Away—
A Dance Step Forward

I was a ballerina. I quit after I injured a groin muscle. It wasn't mine. —**Rita Rudner**

If you can't sing and the only musical instrument you can play is a wooden block, you can certainly dance. The choice of music is yours, from ballroom dancing to frenzy rock, but the advantages of shimmying away your rejection anguish through music are incomparable. Waltzing has the same benefit as working out at a gym.

Doing something physical with your partner forces you to use the motor centers of your brain. According to sex therapist Sallie Foley, "Dancing is the best, outside of sex, because you are always in sync." Health experts are unanimous in suggesting that the perks of tweaking the mind and body through physical involvement in your favorite music will leave you winded, and take the weight off your mind as well as your body.

"How'd you like to dance?" a co-ed asked the young man at the college mixer for new students. "Sorry," said the boy, "but I'm a little stiff from lacrosse." "Look," answered the rejected girl. "I don't care where you're from. I just asked you to dance."

Divine intervention: Joan Wood, only 58, of Sarasota, Florida, went into a tailspin when her husband died. She was financially secure, but she was lonely and retired from her successful public relations business. "I needed a challenge to overcome my depression." So she went to several local dance studios for exercise. Suddenly, her tail-spin life found new wings when her teacher encouraged her to turn exercise into a serious amateur endeavor. She began to travel to dance competitions, and within a few years she became one of the nation's top female dancers in the pro-am category. Now, her life is filled with new friends, who often ask her to give dance exhibitions at small parties. In her mid-70s, she has gotten used to comments like "I don't know how she does it. How old did she say she is?" Her answer is, "The only way you'll find out is if you'll get off your chair and start learning how to dance. Kids, today, don't know what they're missing by not learning ballroom dancing. It's graceful, it's challenging and it's romantic. And you can't beat a combination like that."

Dance your butt off: The TV success of ABC's *Dancing With The Stars* has been a bonanza for dance studios and health clubs that have added dance lessons to aerobic workouts. One club has included lighting and sound systems to their workout room where jazz and ballet are taught. Another teaches belly dancing; another has Indian hip-hop classes, another specializes in two-step country line dancing and many encourage "red hot salsa" and "funky bizness."

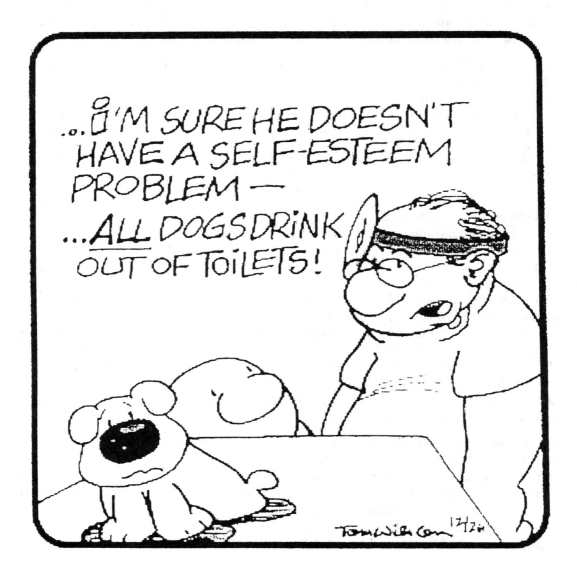

Rub-a-Dub Dub—Relaxing in a Tub

Every guy, when he's nude, looks in the bathroom mirror and thinks he looks substantially better than he is. He figures he's just four or five sit-ups away from being in the hot tub with Pamela Anderson. —**Richard Jeni**

Bare with us: According to a study by the National Women's Health Resource Center, nine of ten adults suffer from stress that could be relieved by warm water therapy. Great for lounging with friends or family, hot tubs provide the following proven physical and mental benefits:

(1) Vasodilatation: They reduce stress, as warm water raises body temperature causing blood vessels to dilate.

(2) Dozy-dotes: Soaking in warm water before bedtime allows sleep to come quicker because of the rise in your body temperature.

(3) Stiff it out: Relief from arthritis and aches results from warm, pulsating water that increases the blood supply to aching joints, thus reducing inflammation. Warm baths have also proven to relieve back and knee pain by reducing stress.

(4) Hot breath: Steam rising from hot water can help open nasal and bronchial passages to improve respiratory health.

(5) Heartfelt: Soaking in hot water has many of the same benefits as exercise, yet places less strain on the heart. It increases the heart rate while it lowers blood pressure.

The Japanese have a word for it: Cypress hot tubs and bathing in hot springs at an *onsen* have been part of Japanese family life for centuries. At spa and meditation gardens, housemaids attend to each guest's outdoor bath settings that include a welcoming cup of tea before and a set dinner after. First they soak you in a streaming pond for a highly ritualized bath, which means scrubbing every pore with a brush, pick, and cloth, then rinsing away any speck of soap, and finally sinking you into a super-heated tub. *Onsen* is not a process you rush through between the ringing of the alarm clock and your first mocha latte. It's about purification and relaxation.

Home, sweet home: Following World War II, thousands of American servicemen brought back to the U.S. not only Japanese culture and sushi, but also proof that bubbling hot spring water is therapeutic for nervous-system disorders as well as muscle damage. Hot tubs, under a brand name like Whirlpool, are now a standard piece of American bathroom installation, and massages by reputable physical trainers are a highlight of every American spa resort. Detractors claim hot tubs are only a short term Band-Aid whose benefits may not last longer than 24 hours. Ah, but then, the hot tub is available tomorrow, too.

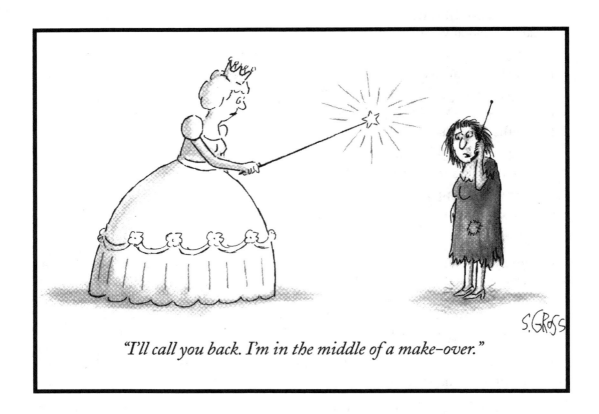

"I'll call you back. I'm in the middle of a make-over."

Hey, Look Me Over—Getting a Make-Over

I don't plan to grow old gracefully. I plan to have facelifts until my ears meet.
—Rita Rudner

A no thin situation: You should never get into a fight you can't win. A perfect example is the fight to stay beautiful. There are demonstrable advantages that accrue to the beautiful—and they are all obvious. From Ponce de Leon to Elizabeth Arden, the hunt for the Fountain of Youth has been a frustrating disappointment and a scam. *New York Times* reporter Alex Kuzynski not only interviewed beautiful people, she wanted to look like one. She was surrounded by people who believed that the face and the body are like a garden, needing to be tended and cared for every day. So she tried to remake herself through plastic surgery. She got Botox injections to remove her smile lines and had liposuction on her thighs and butt. A few years later she had fat removed from her eyelids, and everything else about her—from her hair to her nails—was cosmetically enhanced. But then she finally realized that no one interesting is perfect. She said. "I don't want to sound syrupy, but as Alexander Pope suggested, to err is human, but to forgive ourselves for our imperfections is divine." The psychological problem with cosmetic surgery is that even a transformation to a stunning beauty might not eliminate the memories of the pain of rejection when you felt plain.

I don't need liposuction. I'm just retaining water. Right now, I'm retaining Lake Erie.
—Tom Hodges

A Stone's throw away: For $600, Rita Hazen can change your life from dark to bright. Clients have made her the most sought-after (and expensive) hair colorist in the country. "A lot of women do this after a failed relationship," she claims. "They want to feel sexy and in control of their own lives." Britney Spears wanted something dramatic after filing for divorce, so Hazen created a new hair color that made her look blonder and bolder. "Hey, I'm Britney. I'm back!" she shouted on the David Letterman's *Late Show,* and the crowd roared approval. Everyone at some point considers a change, because staying stagnant is worse. When she was in her 30s, Sharon Stone was the hottest actress in Hollywood. But after 15 glamorous years, Stone became a shining example of the adage that bad luck comes in threes. By the time she was close to 50, major roles evaporated as age faded her sensuous beauty. She anguished over another failed marriage, and she suffered through a life-threatening brain operation. Her major decision was to "use it or lose it." She underwent plastic surgery that kept her from withering on the wine. She accepted small roles and found work playing a western gunslinger, a death row inmate, an ice princess, a Greek muse, an alcoholic wife of a horse breeder, and a beautician. "I had the best," she said, "Now, I'm helping fight African poverty and promoting Middle East peace. We are in a time of odd repression and if popcorn movies allow us to create a platform for celebrity involvement in philanthropy, my life will have had its greatest meaning."

When considering whether or not to have a metal stud put through your tongue, your belly button or your genitalia, take lightning into account. **—Dennis Miller**

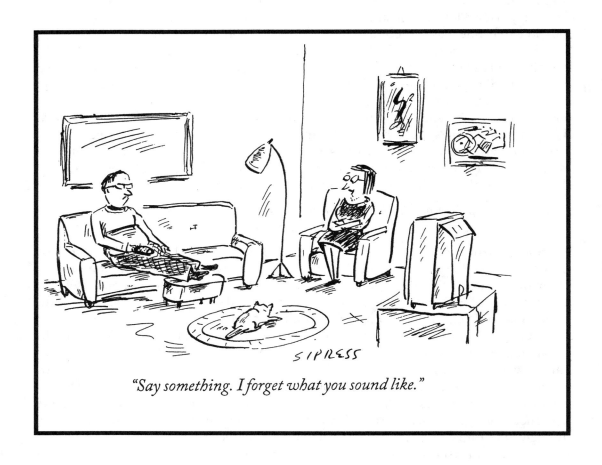

"Say something. I forget what you sound like."

Away With Words—
Giving 'Em the Silent Treatment

My wife and I don't get along. I take my meals separately. I take a separate vacation. I sleep in a separate bedroom and I never talk to her. I'm doing everything I can to keep this marriage together.

Silence may be golden in literature, but the pain of being ignored is right up there with having a proctoscopic procedure. According to Barton Goldsmith of the Scripps Howard News Service, it is appropriate to criticize a behavior but not a person, so the "silent treatment" accomplishes both without an in-your-face accusation. In a personal relationship, if a silence lasts longer than 20 minutes, the defender will start getting anxious. If it lasts for days, a strong message is conveyed, until one party takes the initiative to say, "I don't like the way I'm feeling. Let's talk." If it lasts longer than a few days, eventually Mount Vesuvius will erupt, so prepare to evacuate.

Wear a smile and you have friends; wear a scowl and you have wrinkles. —George Eliot

Smile, baby: It may seem superficial, but the strongest and most impressive silent statement you can make is to just smile. Charlie Chaplin wrote "Smile," a song with lyrics that predict:

Smile though your heart is aching.
Smile even though it's breaking.
When there are clouds in the sky,
You'll get by—if you'll just smile.

Cloudless: Although you can impress people with a Rolex on your wrist or a Jaguar in your garage, a smile is the least expensive way to make you look wise. People think you know the answers when a problem bubbles up. Or, since you don't have problems of your own, that you're much more sympathetic listening to theirs. The major downside is the line, "Hey, what's so funny? This is serious!"

Let a smile be your umbrella, and you'll end up with a pretty soggy hairdo.

Never let 'em see you cry: George Foreman was black, poor and semi-literate. He never read a book until he was fifteen. He was in constant trouble with the law, and he didn't have many possessions. But the two possessions he did have was a boxer's pulverizing jab and a smile that earned him more fans than just winning the heavyweight championship. His championship belt is long gone, but his smile symbolizes a financially successful businessman. He's happy. "I never let my children see me sad," he said. "Children need to feel they can depend on their parents. When you look worried, they get scared. Every time I'm in front of the public or a camera, I smile and laugh. The world is really a great place and my smiling makes it that much better. Keep your smile; it will be your health."

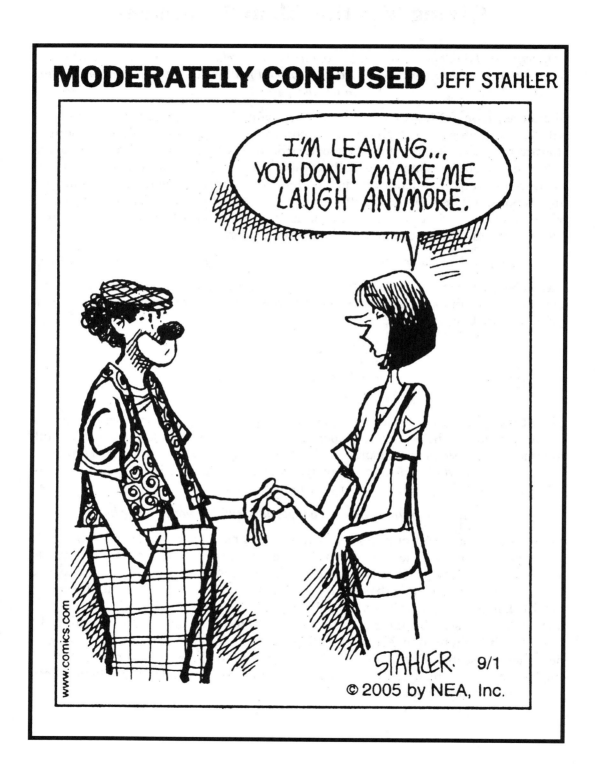

Wit-craft—Using Self-Deprecating Humor

*There is one insult which no human will endure—the assertion that he hasn't a sense of humor. —**Sinclair Lewis***

Beat 'em to the punch: Self-deprecating humor is one of comedy's most popular techniques. If you fear rejection because of some physical, religious, or mental attribute, put yourself down first. Your opponents will often swallow the caustic remarks gagging in their throat. Jimmy Durante became popular by kidding his large proboscis. Kirstie Alley got endorsement deals from diet product sponsors because of her weight problem. Jay Leno kids his chin, and Bob Hope kidded his ski jump nose.

*When I play golf, people keep asking me for my handicap, so I remind them I'm black, I have one eye, I'm five feet tall and I'm Jewish. Isn't that enough? —**Sammy Davis, Jr.***

Old jokes home: Once you get people laughing, you can sell them anything. "Humor is an underutilized tool in the arsenal of crisis communication," wrote Mark S. Katz, a former speechwriter for President Clinton. "It's about solving problems." Anecdotes permit you to exaggerate the details. As a teenager, Billy Crystal was dumped by his girlfriend and his father died—all within 36 hours. "Friends would come over to talk to me, but nobody knew what to say. But suddenly, just when I didn't seem to care about life any more, I heard laughter coming from my family. My crazy Uncle Berns was making everyone laugh with his impersonations. I learned that even in the worst pain, it's okay to laugh. And that's when I decided to be a comedian."

Wit's End: Mark Curry starred in the TV sitcom *Hanging with Mr. Cooper* for five years, but a devastating accident turned his life and material into national prominence. While doing laundry, he knocked an aerosol can into the pilot light of a heater. The explosion engulfed him in flames that burned 18 percent of his body. Despite his crippling pain, he was able to call 911. What surprised him was that to keep from passing out, he kept joking with the operator. "What kind of a fire was it?" she asked. "A hot one!" "And where are you burned?" "Look, does it really make a difference whether it's my leg or my knee. Just get the fuck here!" Now, Curry goes on stage and kids about accidents, being in a coma and contemplating suicide. Funny he should say that.

*Rejection? Who doesn't get it? If the experience is painful, don't block it out. Save it. In three or four days it'll be funny." —**Garry Marshall***

Forgiveness in small packages: I've written hundreds of TV commercials. But there's one I wish I could write, except no American network censor would clear it. It shows a harried father chasing an obnoxious, screaming five-year-old son up and down a supermarket aisle as the terrified boy knocks over displays, sends mountains of food cartons flying in every direction and maliciously pushes shopping carts into little old ladies. The father looks hopelessly at the angry customers, says "Forgive me," and then points to the three-line lettering on his sweat shirt which reads, "Next Time / I'll Use a / Condom."

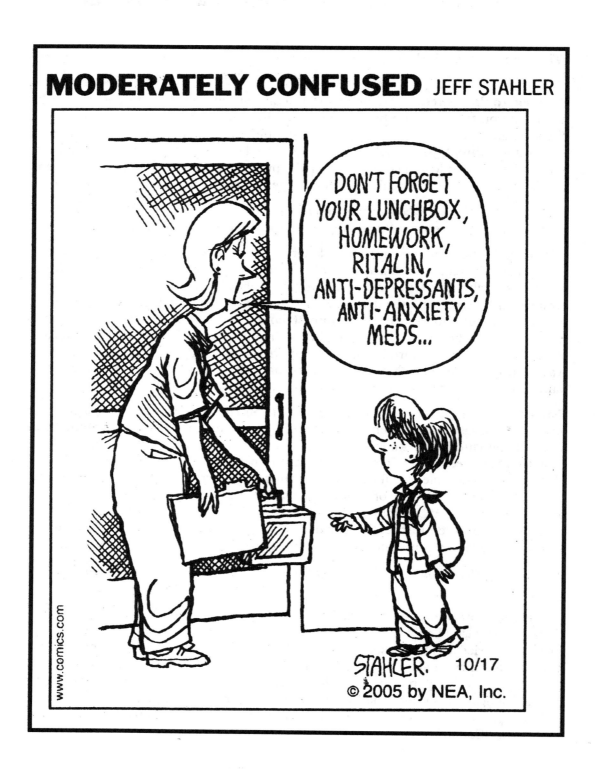

Fixer-Uppers—Taking Daily Medication

Why the controversy about drug testing? There are plenty of guys who'd be willing to test any drug they can come up with. —**George Carlin**

Edgar Allan Prozac: There is no more common first aid for every rejection incident than a dash to the medicine cabinet. When the biggest expansion of the Medicare program in 40 years began in 2006, it lowered prescription costs by as much as 50 percent. Seniors and other eligible beneficiaries stopped running north of the border to buy discount drugs and started demanding prescription medication from their doctors to relieve depression. Sales sky-rocketed. While painkillers, even if taken properly, have a good track record of decreasing anxiety, they are not trouble-free. Common over-the-counter drugs like Ibuprofen can create cardiovascular, gastrointestinal and skin problems. According to a new study, ketamine can cure depression in a matter of hours.

In pain-relieving ingredients, everybody wants extra-strength. They say, "Give me the maximum allowable human dosage. Figure out what will kill me, and then back it off a little bit." —**Jerry Seinfeld**

Good grief: Another concern is the antipsychotic medications frequently prescribed for seniors to treat agitation as well as more serious delirium and dementia. According to Peter Robbins, a professor of psychiatry, "The drugs are overused, even when non-drug approaches would likely be just as beneficial."

Doing what comes naturally: One of the most effective supplements to prescribed medications is not vitamins. It's the natural act of breathing. Proper breathing can increase your state of well-being and release stress. When ABC-TV's Joan Lunden came to Ohio University to interview me for a *Good Morning America* segment, she told me how focused breathing was one of the most effective ways of calming her down when something went wrong in her stressful on-camera, minute-by-minute daily job.

First listen: One of the first training techniques is to listen to your breathing. You'll notice how quickly a conscious breathing technique relaxes your whole body and, within five minutes, a peaceful calm comes over you. "In a crisis, my breath naturally becomes shallow," said Lunden, "and as soon as I notice it, I become more panicked until my mind is out of control. Now, having learned that conscious breathing is a great antidote, I focus on my breath as I inhale and exhale and on how the flow of air feels as it moves through my nostrils." The technique works because your mind cannot concentrate on more than one thought at a time. Placing your total attention to breathing permits you to think, "I'm breathing in serenity. I'm inviting healing into my body."

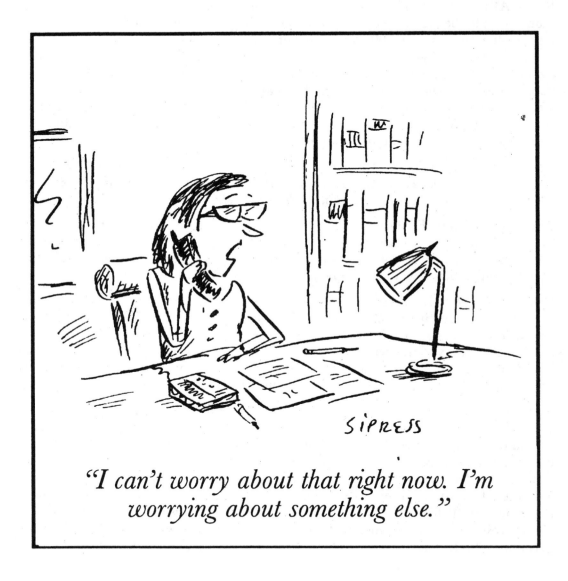

"I can't worry about that right now. I'm worrying about something else."

Do the Trite Thing—Buying Some Time

"I couldn't wait for success, so I went ahead without it." **—Jonathan Winters**

Times up: Respites are respectable. Don't answer a negative remark or a rejection letter immediately. If it's verbal, say "I'll think it over and get back to you." If it's written, let a few days go by before deciding the next action. Then sandwich your reply between compliments that start off with, "Your friendship (or opinion) means a lot to me" and ends with "I look forward to working with you (or sharing our friendship) even more closely in the future." Never let a day end without your having complimented somebody. It's not a coincidence that workers who receive praise on the job have better safety records than those who are angry or depressed.

There should be a giant clock on the top of the Leaning Tower of Pisa. After all, what good is the inclination if you don't have the time?

Site and insight: A university student of mine, Troy Hammond, who became blind at an early age, has become a very successful stand-up comedian. He was able to see the world in a new way—one that surprised (the essence of humor) and delighted his audience. He pointed out that there were many benefits to being blind, such as the ability to decide the beauty of an individual (from their voice), the cleanliness of a room (the delight of every college student), or the absence of fear of the dark (his electric utility was frequently at a loss as to why his monthly bill was so meager). Turning out the lights and contemplating the ways you can solve stress in your life can help eliminate many extraneous elements from the equation of your problem.

Amazing glaze: According to Bernie S. Siegel, in his book *101 Exercises for the Soul,* "resetting your circuit breakers, after a period in the dark, can also reset your desires, expectation, and sense of gratitude." Arthur Sulzberger, Jr., who is now publisher of the *New York Times,* felt lost and insecure at the age of 16 when his parents divorced and he was shuttled between two homes. He was guided to Outward Bound, where mentors put students alone in the wilderness to teach self-reliance. "It taught me to handle adversity. Now, whenever I find myself being bounced around, I can quickly find my center and the truth about myself."

The term "second best" is a misnomer. *Rolling Stone* magazine, in a story about my humor class at Ohio University, called me "the funniest professor in the country." From that day on, my life was miserable. Hundreds of students said, "You're not the funniest. I had a biology teacher who was funnier." Which, of course, is true because biology teachers not only dissect frogs and rabbits, but are also the first to tell co-eds whether or not they're pregnant. So then my publicist started billboarding me as "the second funniest professor in the country." Since no one in America wants to be rated "second best," everyone leaves me alone.

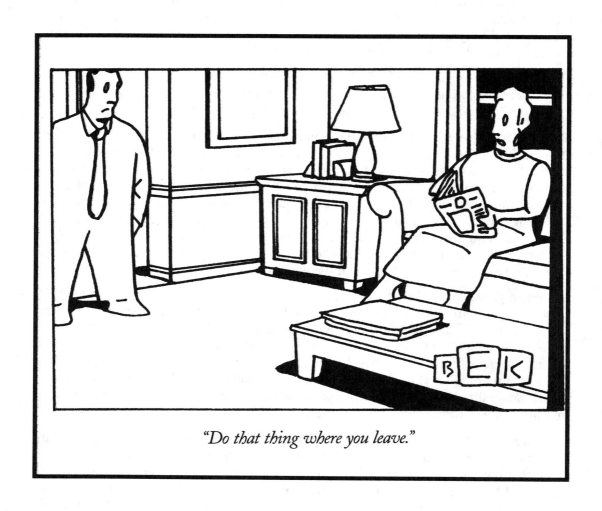

"Do that thing where you leave."

Don't Go Away Mad, Just Go Away—
Controlled Separation

The hardest thing about being dumped in a relationship is listening to songs about being in love or being heartbroken. The only group I was comfortable with was Peter, Paul and Mary when they sang, "If I had a hammer." **—Ellen DeGeneres**

Time out: It's O.K., as part of a healthy relationship, to be alone for a time, even from your spouse or family. That's why a new approach to therapy that is gaining adherents is "controlled separation," a temporary pause on the road to divorce. While one of the individuals agrees to move out of the house, both agree not to speak of their troubles to others to avoid incendiary gossip, and they both complete a written contract that covers areas such as child care, pets, and frequency of personal contact. The time-out should last no longer than six months. According to Lee Raffel in her book *Should I Stay or Go,* half the couples in controlled separation still end up divorcing, but the split is far less acrimonious.

My husband and I used to fight about that night out with the guys, but it's not like I was doing it every night. **—Jenny Jones**

Fear-ever grateful: The greatest deterrent to controlled separation is fear. "It is fear that stops us," according to Frances Moore Lappe and Jeffrey Perkins in their book *You Have the Power.* "Fear can make us powerless and shut us down, or it can allow us to discover our power to create the lives and the world we want." In his *2,000-Year-Old Man* comedy album, when Mel Brooks was asked "What was it 2,000 years ago that transported people quickly from one place to another?" the old man answered, "Fear!" Yet the deepest fear is that of losing one another—a fear of disconnection. The happiest among us are the 30 percent with rich friendship networks and a clearly defined purpose to interact with others, while the other seven in ten feel unsettled about their lives.

Irrational crushes, infatuations, or obsessions. Whatever you want to label it, it's important to reach out to others. **—Janeane Garofalo**

Not bluffing: Another example of controlled separation is temporarily changing your location to a distant and dangerous environment. Actor Sean Penn, often characterized as a homicidal internal combustion engine of rage, wild anger, and aggression, takes time off after his film productions to undertake investigative reporting assignments that help him understand people's pain. As a newspaper correspondent, he went to Iraq and Iran, and he became a hero rescuing helpless survivors in the middle of Hurricane Katrina. Penn quotes William Saroyan. "In the time of your life, live so that there shall be no ugliness or death for any life your life touched."

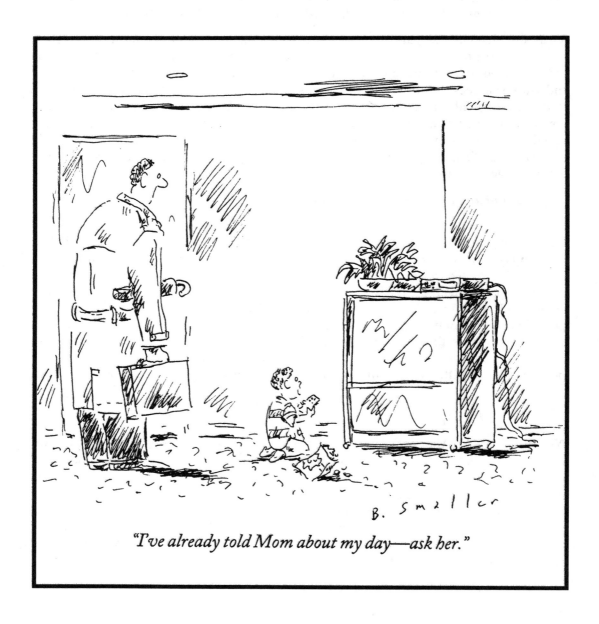

"I've already told Mom about my day—ask her."

Home Alone—Getting to Know the Kids

Why should we put ourselves out for posterity? After all, what has posterity done for us?
—Sir Boyle Roche

Kidding aside: It is acceptable for any person smashed by a major rejection to retreat to family activities that offer an escape from public viewing. Executives often claim that they are retiring—instead of actually being fired—to spend more time with their kids. "It's a guilt that starts the day you are born," says actress Reese Witherspoon. "If you step away from them for two seconds, you immediately feel guilty." These days many will spend more time with their children then they bargained for. According to a Harvard University study four million 25–34 year-old college graduates go back to live with parents.

College senior to friend, "I'm writing a letter begging her to take me back. No, not my girlfriend, my mother!"

No bully for entitlement: For most children, learning to avoid rejection is taught in their preschool years. Schools will not permit in-house parties, even Valentine's Day cards, if invitations aren't given to everyone in class. For kids younger than eight or nine, scorekeeping at soccer or softball games is no longer permitted and every player in the league gets a trophy. Parents are warned that their rejection of a child's modest activity could represent a serious blow to self-esteem that could last for a lifetime. Whether this is wisdom or foolishness depends on the advisor. "Self-esteem comes from a job well done, when you've actually achieved something," said critic Dr. Georgette Constantinou, a pediatric psychiatrist. "How can do expect them to handle life's big bumps if they haven't experienced the little ones?" Kids grow up with an inflated sense of self-worth. "It's always a trophy," said one teacher. "They have no sense that you have to work hard for some things." On the other hand, some child guidance specialists urge parents to find something specific to praise. You can give them an award for being the best helper of the week, best cleaner of the week, or the happiest person of the week. Learning to compete—even for minor awards—teaches them to develop their skills.

Resilience: There are few more devastating rejections that getting a terminal illness. That's what actor Michael J. Fox discovered when he was diagnosed with Parkinson's disease. His greatest sense of strength and reassurance, he said, is not his medications but his family. "I get to spend a lot of time with my kids, which few parents do. I know what each of them is doing in school, who their friends are, what's happening with their activities." With his illness in front of them, he doesn't have to hammer them with lectures on doing things in spite of challenges. "I set my children an example just by being there. You know you have great kids, when they think you're still funny."

Emptynestrogen is a new suppository that eliminates loneliness by reminding you how awful your kids were as teens and how you couldn't wait till they moved out.

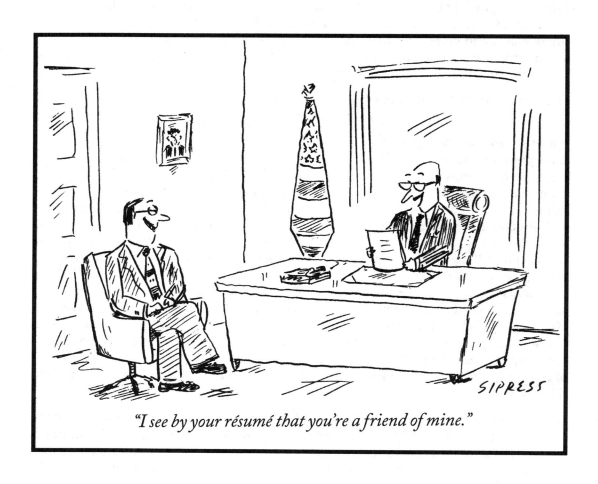

"I see by your résumé that you're a friend of mine."

Home Court Advantage—
Retreating to a Project

My wife said to me, "All you do with your spare time is sit around and drink beer. You need a hobby." So I got a hobby. I make beer. —**Dave Barry**

Sharing her gift: Invariably every celebrity selects one major charity to endorse. Halle Berry didn't need to choose. Diabetes selected her when she discovered she had Type I just as she was carving out her acting career. Rather than accept the disease as a knockout blow, Berry claims that her need to keep her body in shape with diet, exercise, and meditation was a gift. "When I was ten," she reported, "my teacher told me that when I grew up, I was going to be given a gift. Diabetes turned out to be that gift. I raise money for research, but learning to deal with the disease has given me the toughness I need for an exhausting career that recently produced an Academy Award. Diabetes is not funny, but when others frown, I insist upon smiling." Berry has proven that beauty is not skin deep.

To err is human. To blame it on your computer is even more so. —**Robert Orben**

To write a wrong: Some of the most beneficial major retreats are creative writing or fine arts courses at a local college, or family endeavors like hiking or camping. When David Paterson was eight, his best friend was killed by lightning while the two of them were camping. Feeling guilty, he begged his mother, an author, to write a children's book that would make sense of his anguish. With his help, she did, and her award-winning novel *Bridge to Terabithia* was also a popular film. "Writers write to survive as individuals," claims Anna Quindlen. "Writing can make pain tolerable and confusion clearer." There's also something to be said for walking behind a gas engine lawn mower for solitude. The noise will drown out your anger.

Caveman to friend playing golf, "I feel safe in saying that this game we've invented will be a calming and soothing influence on mankind for all time to come."

One step at a time: If you wish to be alone for a while, hiking is a perfect physical activity, but take a dog along who has learned how to lick your hand. Joe Lawson's father committed suicide when he was 16. He felt trapped by depression, but he was too ashamed to ask for help. Joe learned that depression was an illness that can be treated, so to help focus world attention to Expedition Hope, an organization that sponsors treatment of depression, he undertook the most arduous feat in mountain climbing: scaling the seven highest summits, the highest in each continent. At the peak of each summit, Joe places a photo of his father and himself. "If I'm going to do this," he said, "I might as well do it for a good cause." He claims there is a parallel between depression and mountain climbing. Both are long, hard struggles that must be conquered one step at a time. "The summit is always reachable, no matter how difficult."

Wife to husband, "You say you want to walk in the moonlight. Sounds like a great idea, so take the dog with you."

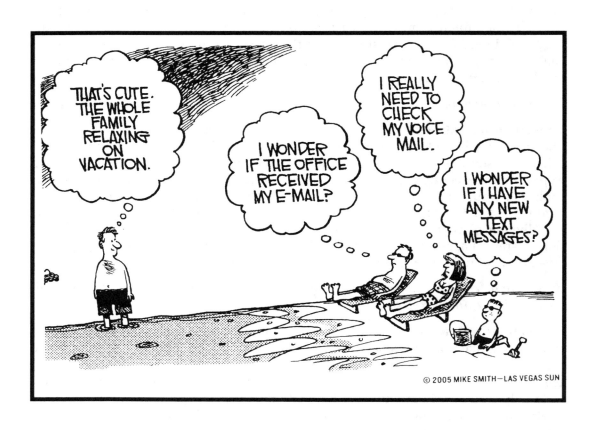

Don't Resist a Rest—Taking a Vacation

They say the typical symptoms of stress are eating too much, smoking too much, drinking too much, impulse buying and driving too fast. Are they kidding? That's my idea of a great day. —**Monica Piper**

Take a vacation when you go on vacation: Go somewhere. It's good medicine. A vacation has therapeutic value. It refreshes you and makes you more creative. Since stress is the body's natural response to day-to-day external events, make time to get away from it all, but don't let your red badge of courage get packed in your luggage. It doesn't have to equal one of Homer's odysseys, but it should be a trip that is activity driven and not just a cabin in the woods or a cottage by the shore. As pleasant as the latter choices appear, they provide too much opportunity to keep regurgitating the original rejection. "If hitting the road sounds like avoidance," says clinical psychologist Thomas Demaria, "sometimes not facing something can help people gain perspective and allows them to heal." As each day goes by, you'll start emptying your mental suitcase of dirty laundry. You will be increasing your total energy, not just evaluating your total life style. The first few days are rarely that beneficial, so to be truly refreshed the amount of time away should last at least a month and even six months may not be too long to fully revitalize the spirits. By that time the public has forgotten what all your fuss was about, even if your spouse hasn't.

Sleepless in Seattle: According to Pauline Wallin, author of *Taming Your Inner Brat: A Guide for Transforming Self-Defeating Behavior,* part of our narcissist culture is the feeling that things won't go right if you take time off. Research indicates that death by heart disease is 40 percent higher in people who shun vacations. Joyce Gannon of the *Pittsburgh Post-Gazette* advises, "Keep that tech-savvy laptop and cell phone at home."

Getting whacked: Don't ask yourself every vacation day, "What do I really want out of life?" Stress disorder and obsessive-compulsive disorder are marked by angst that is out of whack with reality, claims Erin Bried.

Leave old baggage behind. The less you carry, the further you go. —**Allen Klein**

Margaret Loftus of *National Geographic* recommends challenging yourself with a trip with a foreign language. "It's hard to think of anything else when you're negotiating a purchase with someone who doesn't speak English." Bring back souvenirs to jog your memory for years after. When you do return home, it will be with a stronger strength of self. You'll have control and your life back.

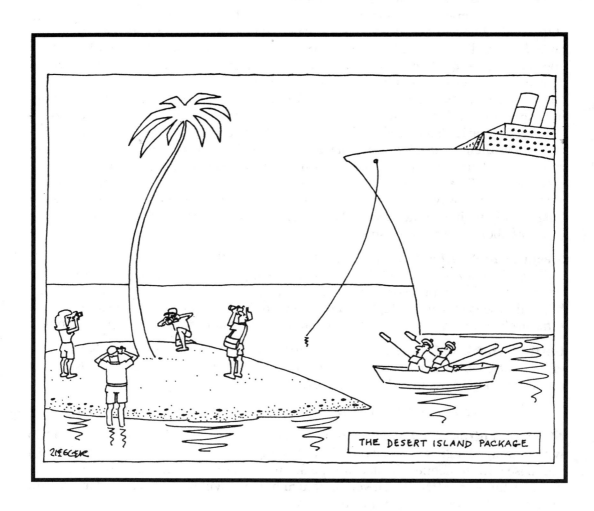

THE DESERT ISLAND PACKAGE

Yachts of Fun—
The Month-Long Getaway Cruise

Last year, my husband and I took a trip around the world. This year, we're going somewhere else.

Don't rush it: Our minds and bodies are closely intertwined. It takes four to six weeks to repair a broken bone and it takes four to six weeks to heal a broken heart.

Give me a cruise with sunshine, fresh air, great food and a beautiful, sexy partner, and you can keep the sunshine, food and fresh air. —Jack Benny

She's still a virgin: If you can afford it, there is no better getaway therapy than a month-long cruise on a private yacht. The latest multi-million-dollar super yachts have made cruising the Mediterranean, the Caribbean, or the South Pacific the choice of sea-lebrities who nickname it a C-worthy escape. Some of the yachts are equipped with a movie theater, a concert hall, and a full recording studio. Others have tiled swimming pools that rise at night to become dance floors. You can go deep-sea fishing, tour the underworld in a miniature submarine, play cards, work on your golf swing, get daily massages, and, on one cruise, even take a daily champagne shower.

We wanted to do some international traveling last summer, but the State Department warned us that if we wanted to hear a foreign language, we should go only to places that love America. So we ended up in Cleveland. —Mel Helitzer

Jamaica me tan: A yacht's high-end service has become fashionable not only to get to foreign ports but also to have invitations to major local events and dinner parties to meet VIP movers and shakers who live there. These customized matchmaking services are not for the general public. They cost thousands of dollars, but travel agents can arrange everything from private jets to presidential suites to finding a new soul mate. When you return home, it will be with a stronger appreciation of what you have in the United States. You'll have your life back.

Europe is terrific. If you go there, don't miss it.

It's all there: You can find a monthly update on available cruises and tour operators in the Emporium section of Travel + Leisure magazine. If you plan on traveling alone, the book *The Practical Nomad: How to Travel Around the World* could be helpful. There are also workshops for women traveling solo, the web site www.Journeywoman.com, and the book *Go Girl! The Black Woman's Book of Travel Adventure,* which offers information for women of any race. And if this kind of pandering doesn't cure your depression, there's always the next page.

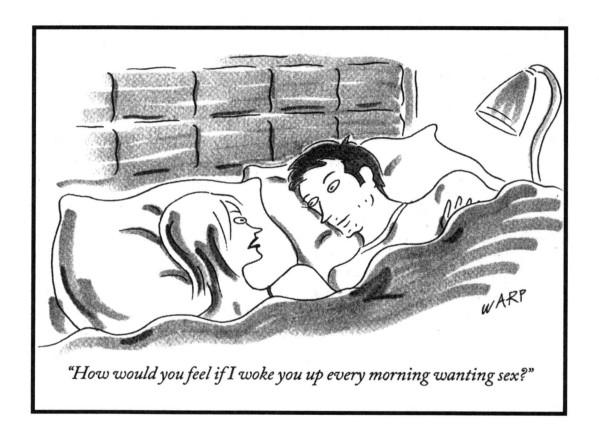

"How would you feel if I woke you up every morning wanting sex?"

Viagra Falls—Sex and Love

The difference between love and sex is that sex relieves tension and love causes it.
—Woody Allen

Nothing risqué, nothing gained. Love is an inlet and sex is an outlet. For example, writers' libidos are stimulated when they get a rejection slip. According to J.O. Bromfield, 77 percent of writers researched had orgasmic sexual activity within 24 hours following receipt of a rejection slip. While common advice is that you should never become committed to anyone on the rebound, becoming involved in a new romance after rejection is solid advice because of the time and energy required. As Cole Porter wrote in his song "Night and Day":

> *Whether near to you or far*
> *It makes no difference, darling, where you are*
> *I think of you, night and day.*
> *In the roaring traffic boom*
> *In the silence of my lonely room*
> *I think of you, night and day.*

Up at the count of five: There are five essential basic building blocks to start a serious friendship:

(1) Speak the name often,
(2) Be tactile (a handshake, an embrace, and touching the arm or shoulder),
(3) Smile often,
(4) Say "thank you" after every positive action,
(5) Offer compliments at every opportunity without seeming superficial.

Women need to feel loved to have sex, and men need to have sex to feel loved. How did we ever get started? —Billy Connolly

Bulk male: As an outlet for rejection, few actions are more mentally and physically exhausting than the pursuit of sex because it requires long-term mental scheming and physical gyrations, at least on the part of men. The taboo blanket that was once over pre-marital sex is no longer saleable, and the popularity of such TV programs as *Sex in the City* and *Desperate Housewives* prove that woman are as desirous of sexual frolicking as are men.

A survey asked married women when they most want to have sex. 84 percent said right after their husband is finished. —Jay Leno

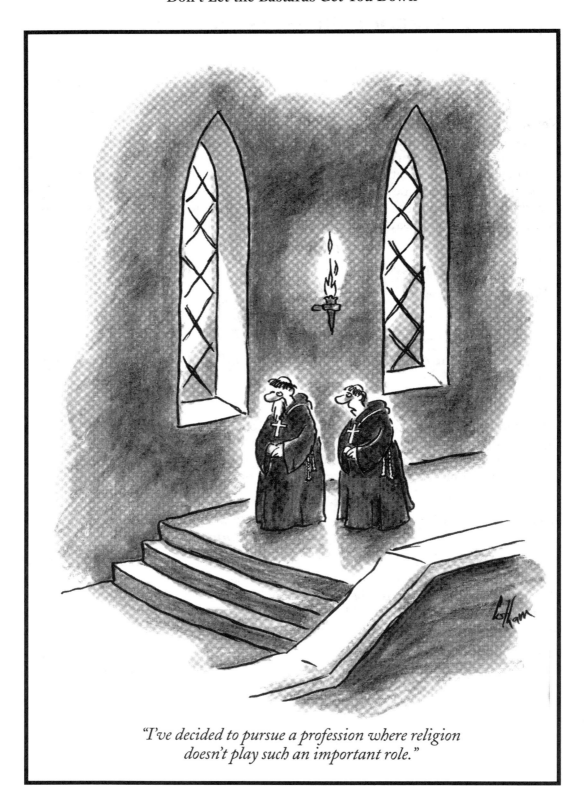

"I've decided to pursue a profession where religion doesn't play such an important role."

Pray Tell—Nearer Your God to Thee

More than any time in history, mankind faces a crossroads. One path leads to despair and utter helplessness. The other leads to extinction. Let us pray that we have the wisdom to choose correctly. —**Woody Allen**

Parish the thought: Even though religion is taking its lumps these days with the Catholic clergy being degraded by child molestation cases, and the Ten Commandments being bounced from courthouse lobbies, you still have to put your hand on a Bible when you're being sworn in court, and our coins still are embossed "In God We Trust." Retreating to religious devotions, such as praying, reading the Bible, and seeking guidance from your spiritual leader, is still a popular method for overcoming rejection. "Just remember," said Apostle Brian S. Lewis, "Jesus was the most rejected man who ever lived."

Now I believe we should all treat each other like Christians. I will not, however, be responsible for the consequences. —**George Carlin**

Revelation: Recent surveys indicate that more than 90 percent of the general public believes in the existence of a supreme being, while only 10 percent of leading scientists still do. But science works best in the brain, while religious faith works best in the heart. Science doesn't attempt to explain your ethics or your self-respect, even if it does provide a lot of footnotes. When you are uncertain how to deal with disappointment, claims Pastor Lynn Miller, you need to look beyond yourself to the God of your faith. "By turning to God," she says, "you will hear words of assurance that you are indeed loved. God is big enough to handle whatever you feel, as in the 23rd Psalm: "The Lord is my shepherd, I shall not want—even though I walk in the darkest valley, I fear no evil for you are with me."

A room with a pew: When you are searching for your own moral compass, you should use every available avenue, including a God to whom one may pray in expectation of receiving an answer. Like if he created everything in six days, why was he in such a hurry? In 1996, eight years before he ran for U.S. Vice President, John Edwards' son Wade was killed in an auto accident. He and his wife, Elizabeth, were overtaken with grief. Even with strangers, she would take out Wade's picture and tell them about her son. "It made some people feel awkward, but I was always sure to say how much it meant that they would listen." She found the most solace in going to his grave every day and reading aloud from the Bible. "It only was there," she said, "that I could speak to him."

God fearing or God loving: Rather than accusing God of failing you, religious counseling can minimize your problem through prayer and reading the Bible. Not all religions encourage forgive and forget, but all of them encourage you to heal yourself by putting God first in your life.

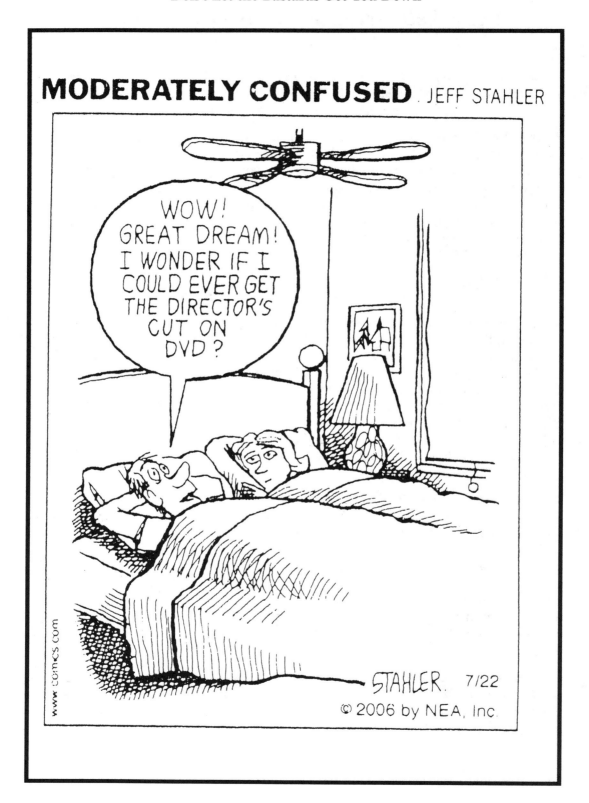

Go Gently Into the Night—
To Sleep, Perchance to Dream

You're the writer, director and producer of your own dreams. **—Lincoln Navigator ad**

Beddy-bye: One of the best remedies for a case of rejection is to get a good night's sleep. The old adage is right. Things really do look better in the morning. But getting into bed and staying there is also an escape that's been used by celebrities. Aaron Spelling holds the record as the world's most prolific and richest TV producer. He had almost 200 productions, including miniseries like *Charlie's Angels* and *Fantasy Island* that ran for years on ABC network. Yet, when his final production was canceled, Spelling was so distraught that he took to his bed (in the largest home in Hollywood) and refused to get out for weeks. Many say his emotional distress contributed to the stroke that caused his death.

Depressed people, unless they sleep a lot, are cruel. **—Renata Adler**

Sound a sleep: The amount of sleep you need depends on age, lifestyle, genetics, and what you did the night before. It's easier to shut off the light than it is to shut off your head. When you're stressed, you may go to bed later in the night, which makes you feel tired the next day. Then, if you're grouchy during the day, it's O.K. to sneak in a nap. Teens need nine hours of sleep, while adults feel fine with seven or eight hours.

Dreaming permits us to be quietly and safely insane every night. **—William Dement**

Timing is important, too: If you don't fall asleep within five minutes of lying down, you are probably sleep deprived or may even suffer from a sleep disorder. Coffee, alcohol, and smoking can affect the quality of your sleep. Give up these vices, and you improve not only the quality of your sleep, but end up needing less. While regular exercise is beneficial, you should end your physical exercise three hours before bedtime.

When I woke up this morning, my girlfriend asked me, "Did you sleep well?" I said, "No, I made a few mistakes." **—Steven Wright**

Double or nothing: Insomnia is not uncommon in a world of 24/7 workdays, jetlag and a growing dependency on pills. Nearly 35 million prescriptions for sleep medication were filled in 2006, a number doubling every five years. While current medications are not as miraculous as advertising suggests, they are superior to barbiturates, which are deadly when mixed with alcohol. Moreover, research does not support traditional claims that listening to soft music, reading a vapid book, spraying pillow mist, using ylang-ylang lotions, or wearing an eye mask have any long-term benefit. But no pill works as well as sex. But we've said that before—and we will again.

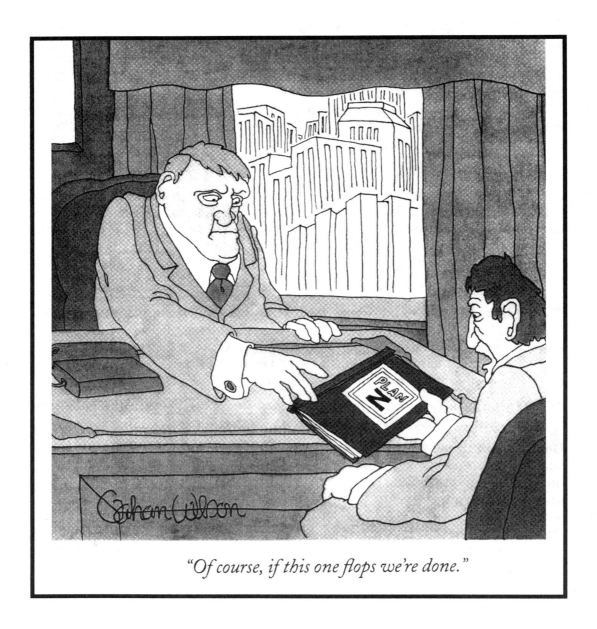

"Of course, if this one flops we're done."

Experiment—Finding a New Goal

Be curious
Though interfering friends may frown
Get furious at each attempt to hold you down
If this advice you'll always employ
The future can offer you infinite joy
And merriment, experiment, then you'll see
—Cole Porter

A leg down: Goals help you become an achiever. And goal seekers—not goal keepers—are happiest when they are making progress, instead of feeling trapped in a situation where stagnation is all they can anticipate. Bob Kerrey is a university president, deciding when to run for President again. He is a Medal of Honor hero who lost his leg in Vietnam, as well as being a former governor and later two-term senator from Nebraska. His first Presidential try, in 1992, was a failure as a result of an unfortunate lesbian joke during a newspaper interview that was captured on tape. Though he spent agonizing days apologizing, nothing could extract him from his personal "tunnel of horrors." He believes, "You've got to really want to be President. You've got to have a passion for it. You can't be entirely happy if you walk away from your goal because of the possibility of failure."

My strength lies solely in my tenacity. **—Louis Pasteur**

A body of work: No case history could be more intuitively inspiring than that of Thomas Quasthoff, a thalidomide victim, who stands four feet four inches tall, on stumpy legs without knee joints or much thigh. His hands emerge from his shoulders like flippers. Despite a youth spent in institutions for the severely handicapped, he refused to sulk, studied music as a way to boost his spirits, and today is one of the world's most famous lieder singers. "I was depressed for a long time, constantly lonely and shut out of music schools because I could not physically play a piano. I worked hard to demonstrate to myself—as well as others—that birth defects will not prevent me to get anything I really want." A *New York Times* critic agreed. "Before a sold out audience, even before he utters a sound, he turns his head and with a wide smile that is both beatific and earthy, wins over the crowd in an instant."

Most men lead lives of quiet desperation. **—Henry David Thoreau**

Be different or die: According to Dr. Allen Fox, a former nationally ranked tennis player, participating in sports trains athletes to select a roadmap of three essential steps in the goal formula. They work for non-athletes, too:

(1) Identify a specific goal (like winning) that is attainable and logical.

(2) Select short bite-sized action projects that are measurable along the way.

(3) Go for the pot of gold with everything you can afford.

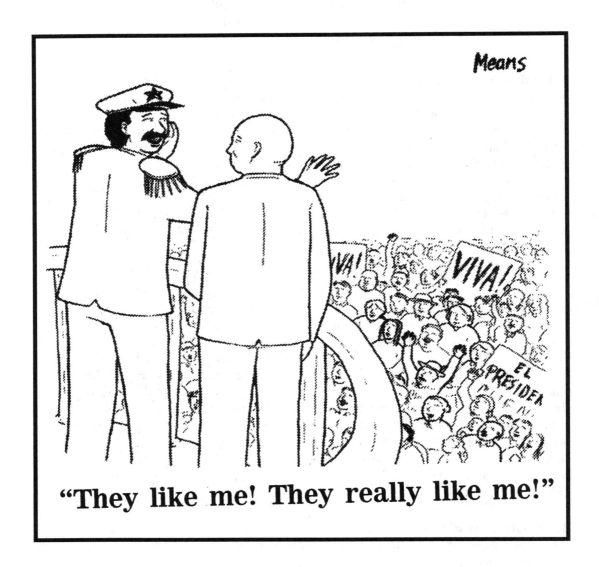

Follow Me—Being a Leader

Whenever I was asked to do something gutsy, I'd say "yes," and then I'd figure out how to do it. —Joan Lunden

Find heroes: One person can make a difference. A leader is dedicated to action, not to excuses, those little deaths that read like a detailed obituary. Nothing can be as humiliating as rushing to a hospital emergency room and then being rejected because there were not enough medical personnel or beds available for your treatment. Much of the problem has been funding, and it will take extraordinary leadership to ameliorate the problem. Typical of those leaders fighting a hospital's rejection of patients is Dr. David Sklar, chairman of the University of New Mexico Emergency Medicine Department. Sklar claims: "Emergency rooms have miscalculated what they need for beds, doctors, nurses and technicians. It gets pretty crazy because it takes 12 to 15 hours, sometimes days, to get admitted. Nurses are under so much pressure that they have high burnout and turnover. It shouldn't be that way." If Sklar can help, it won't be.

I'm not a good lover, but at least I'm fast. —Drew Carey

Leadership skills are life skills that develop early in your life. As a result, ordinary people can rise to extraordinary talent. Oprah Winfrey claims she started believing she was special at the age of four when she started being an orator. "Whenever you do something a lot," she said, "you get good doing it." In his biography of Lyndon Johnson, author Robert A. Caro wrote that "all his adult life, because of the agonies of his youth, the insecurity and shame of growing up poor, Johnson grasped frantically at every chance to escape that past, no matter how slender." Biographers most often credited Johnson's successful work ethic as energy, but in fact the only emotion that governed Johnson's life was ambition. Any other emotions, he claimed, were luxuries. Then there are those who believe the best way to cope with managerial stress is to be the one who caused it.

Belle of the ball: If you're a prostitute, pimp, homosexual, drug addict, or gangster and want to be welcome in a religion, then Patti LaBelle's church is waiting to welcome you. Born Patrician Louise Holte in an impoverished area of Philadelphia, the famous singer spends much of her time off the concert stage not only doing humanitarian work for cancer research but also making her church less judgmental and more available to the underdogs of society. "Churches should open up our arms and hearts to all kinds of people. We must love our sisters and brothers and protect them," she claims. "They're living their own lifestyle, but we're all God's children and I will fight until the end for them."

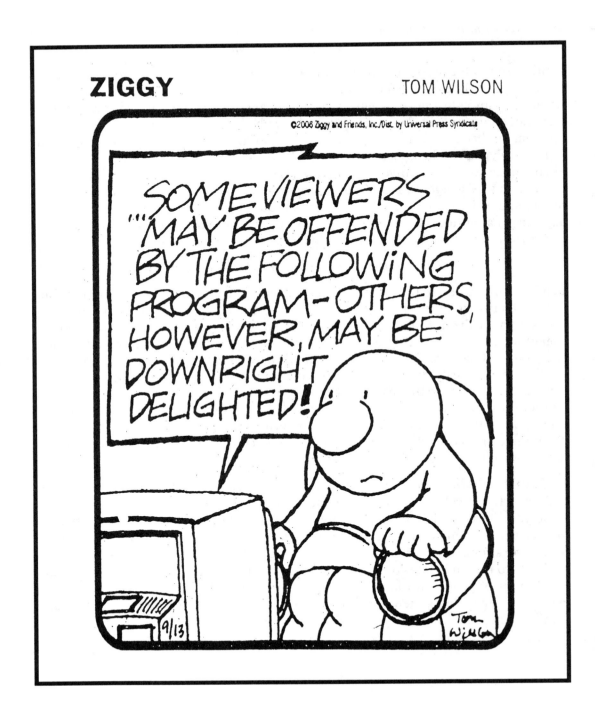

When Half Are Below Average—
Being a Team Player

Lonely people live shorter lives than the general public. —**Alan McGinnis**

The friendship factor: It doesn't have to be a formal team, but by encouraging those around you to join an extensive network of loyal friends ("I'll rub your back, if you'll rub mine!") to achieve some specific goal, you'll also be helping yourself adjust to rejection punches. Social incompetence accounts for 60 to 80 percent of all job failures. According to Richard Farson, professor of humanistic psychology, "Millions of people have never had one minute in their whole lifetime where they could share with another person their deeper feelings."

The casting couch audition: Actress Charlize Theron is as intelligent as she is talented. She claims that she has never suffered the indignities of a casting couch audition, because when she walks into a room, her demeanor sends off an unspoken message that says, "Look, I'm smart. Don't even try to pull one over on me. When I act like that, I never give anyone any inkling that that kind of behavior is even remotely possible."

No cloning allowed: Don't try casting members of your new team in your own image. Just be satisfied if they're loyal. "I can never be satisfied with anyone who would be blockheaded enough to have me," said Abraham Lincoln, a line that was copied by Groucho Marx: "I would never want to be a member of any country club that would have me as a member."

Trust me: By an overwhelming margin, women rate their friends by trust and confidentiality. Men, on the other hand, describe a friend as someone to share an activity. That's why men find it's easier to provide wise counsel and harder to listen and accept it. So don't let pride stand in the way of accepting (or eliciting) advice and help from those around you. Look for ways to contribute your talent and experience to younger "players on the team," and you'll find their help increases geometrically.

Take-over: A small team has tremendous power, and a group of 30 students can dictate policy for the entire university. It's a comparatively easy plan. Each of the students joins every major campus organization and then, by block vote, elects one of their team as president and others to chair influential committees. Then the 30 organizations can issue joint public proclamations, denounce or approve university policy, and even demand the firing of most college administrators. Only delegates from 13 colonies signed the Declaration of Independence. Benjamin Franklin once observed, "We had better all hang together or we will certainly all hang separately."

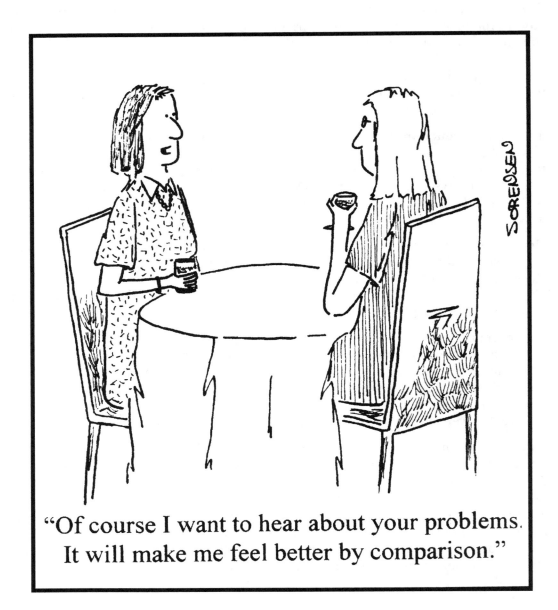

Tip-Toe Thru the Juleps—Let's Take Lunch

When I have lunch with my boss, I always have a problem in ordering. What kind of wine goes with heartburn?

As Job asked: "Why do bad things happen to good people?" That's the thesis of your lunch. As soon as the physical lament of rejection passes, invite your critic to lunch. It is the business world's first wonder drug. Even though disagreement is being discussed, there's something about the mood of confrontation while you're having a meal that changes a hostile confrontation into a social event. It eliminates the formality and quickly scales down the uproar to a manageable discussion. According to Patricia Nelson Limerick, author of *Something in the Soil,* listening and then considering a solution can turn an adversary into a friend.

God gave us one tongue, but two ears. Obviously, he knows something about the value of confrontational negotiation.

Lunch break: Following a broken engagement, Irene LaCota was suddenly single. She tried personal ads, even blind dates on recommendations of friends. Nothing worked. She found single bars dangerous, dating services impersonal and most online chat rooms filled with phony headshots or personal profiles. Then she founded "It's Just Lunch," a dating middleman that arranges first dates that last just an hour. Her service bloomed as clients found that they could actually meet in a relaxed atmosphere and talk without pressure. Her agency is now the fastest growing dating service in the world with more than 100 offices. "I get to do something that can change someone's life in a big way," she gushed.

The pleasure of your company: If your agitator won't come to a lunch, then invite a friend. Only one friend, at most two. The success of a good luncheon conversation depends on politeness, and with three or more guests you're forced to spend a majority of the time listening to their problems. It should be an instrument of impulse and not treated as a thoughtful preparation of analytical research.

Avoid rush hour service. In France, Spain, and Italy, you can linger over a luncheon drink. But in the U.S., casual table service is encouraged only after 2 p.m. You must find a quiet section of the restaurant, which is increasingly difficult. Otherwise, it's likely that the person at the next table will be eating with one hand, holding a cell phone to his ear, fidgeting with a laptop on one side, a TV set in front, tapping his feet to rock music blaring from loudspeakers behind, and yet be visibly annoyed when your private conversation is audible. You need an atmosphere conducive to reflective conversation.

An elderly man was fitted for hearing aids that allowed him to hear 100% for the first time in twenty years. A month later his doctor said, "Your family must be really pleased you can hear again." The man replied, "Oh, they don't know I'm not deaf any more. I just sit at meals and listen to them laugh about me. I've changed my will three times!"

143

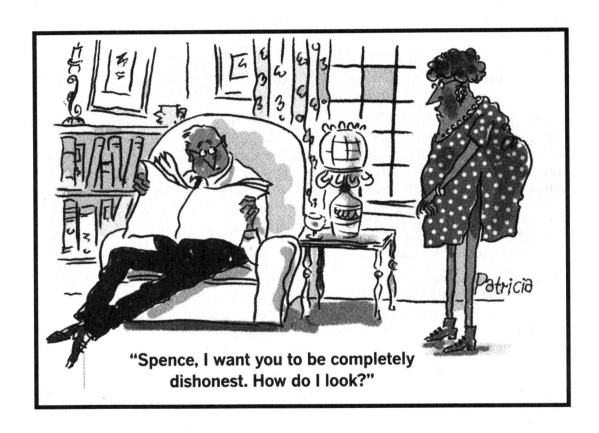

Let's Face It—Putting on a Positive Outlook

I was flying and this guy was sitting next to me and I could tell he really wanted me—to shut up. Because he kept saying, "Shut the fuck up." I'm chatting and chatting, and he's busy flying the plane. And like he's very focused—on that bottle of vodka.
—Wendy Liebman

The pursuit of happiness: A new aspect of therapy is "positive psychology," in which analysts focus on your strengths, on what makes you feel good, and conditions that make you feel happy. "It's about working on your strengths," said Tayyab Rashid, a Toronto psychologist, "and there are no short cuts." Actress Salma Hayek was the idol of her native Mexico, except for one physical characteristic. She is only 5'2" and in Mexico it is very important to be tall. Some say being short is a deformity. For years, her classmates teased her because she was always first in line. "I was very upset," said Salma, "until one day I said, who decided it was better to be tall? Am I less healthy? Am I less capable? I realized it was a dirty trick. Everybody tried to make you fit a standard, and it's based on nothing. So I came to Hollywood where I am viewed as someone beautiful. I have a confidence in myself that a lot of tall girls don't."

Merry missives: The object is that by concentrating on the positive, you will have fewer bad moods. It is not for anyone with a mental illness, but even victims of a disaster can be encouraged to focus on how they survived. "Holocaust suffering confers no privileges," claims Nobel laureate Elie Wiesel. "It's what you do with it." The skill is in finding a *raison d'etre* that is logical and not an obvious scam.

I went to Baghdad to find out what made those Iraqis tick, and I discovered it was a bomb strapped to their chests.

Avoiding avoidance: The producers of *The Cosby Show* were prepared to cancel the weekly taping the day after Bill Cosby's son, Ennis, was murdered. But Cosby insisted that production continue. He did not want to grieve alone. "Whoever took his life is riding with the devil now," he said. Then he commissioned a mahogany bust of his son to stand in the foyer of his home. No one can go into the house without facing it. Each day, Cosby stands directly in front of Ennis' bust and tells him the best news he can learn about his son's friends and siblings. "Nothing can stop you," repeats Cosby. "Nothing can stop you."

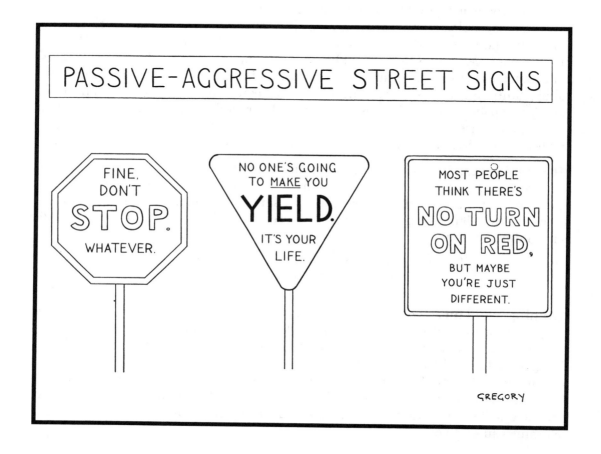

Fools Rush In—Pursuing Multiple Activities

Vacuuming sucks! When I get mad it makes me want to clean. So my wife spends most of the day following me around trying to piss me off. —**Reno Goodale**

The invisible slam: "Don't get mad, don't even try to get even," claims fashion designer Diane von Furstenberg. "Just ignore him. To remain angry at someone, after all, is never to be free of him." And her recourse from rejection is to pursue multiple activities. The DVF woman, her mythical alter ego, is young, beautiful, has many lovers, and a career that makes her independent of men. She is always in control, in business and in romance. She never waits for the phone to ring. The von Furstenberg process is that "When something happens that appears to be bad, it is actually for the best."

I spilled spot remover on my dog. Now, he's gone. —**Steven Wright**

Let me count the ways: Do something different. Temporarily change your daily habits: wear new clothes, change your hairstyle, listen to a different radio or TV station, and take a new route to work. Don't let any one assignment sap all your enthusiasm or energy. Be resilient. Minimize the importance of each event. "It's no big deal." Sometimes simply the chemistry wasn't right. Sometimes your competitors developed the product before you did. Rather than be obstinate, change your focus. Professor John Shank of Dartmouth preaches that the only things in the middle of the road are yellow lines and dead skunks. If you compromise commitment, you end up as flattened road kill.

My wife is into multi-tasking, which means she's usually talking on the phone when we're having sex.

Oprah-licious: When you're one of the most successful women in the world, and you're a famous talk-show diva called Oprah Winfrey, you don't expect to encounter disagreement, let alone rejection. But the belief that whatever Oprah wants, Oprah gets is a myth. All her life, she has faced and overcome hostility, discrimination and major obstacles. She grew up poor—a real coal miner's daughter. As a pre-teen she was raped, discarded by her parents and raised by her grandmother in a home without running water or electricity. She was fired by WJZ-TV in Baltimore as a news anchor because she wasn't suited to TV. Her dream was to build a lavish leadership academy for South Africa's brightest girls who had little hope of an ambitious future, but the government turned down partnership, fearful that the lavish school would be too elitist for such a poor nation. So Oprah went ahead on her own. She poured $40 million of her own money into the project, personally interviewed every finalist candidate for the middle school class, and even selected the architects, the uniforms, the beds, and the china. "I see myself in all these girls," she said. "I understand what it means to grow up not loved. I wanted to be encouraged. I wanted to be inspired. I still feel the pain. This school will be the fulfillment of my work on earth."

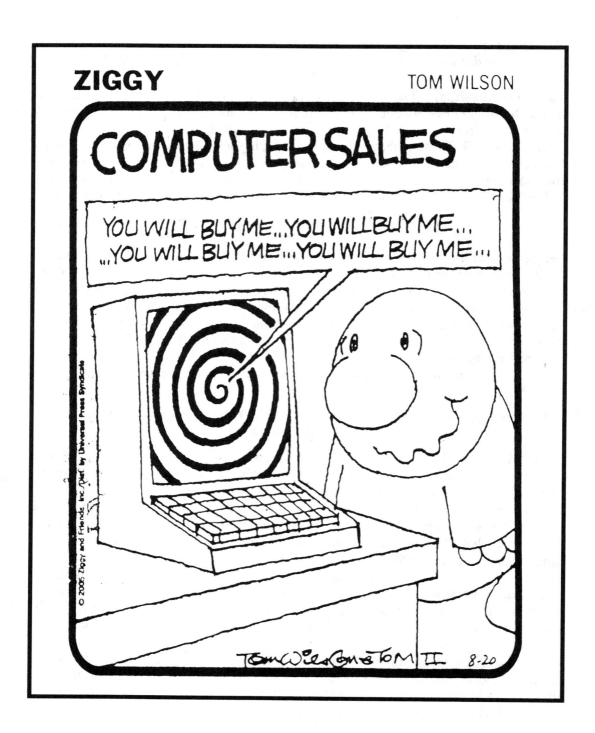

The Wheel of Fortune—Closing the Sale

I'm a writer. I write fiction. Mostly, it's checks. —**Wendy Liebman**

Closing the sale: No matter what your profession or craft, you're always selling something—a product, an idea, or an agreement on action. And rejection is nothing more than one strikeout in your batting average. So the goal is improving that average.

Don't be afraid of missing opportunities. Behind every failure is an opportunity somebody wishes they had missed. —**Lily Tomlin**

Here's the formula:

(1) Believe in what you're selling.
(2) Since most prospects want to like you before they'll agree to buy anything, spend more time in knowing them and understanding their responsibilities.
(3) Find out what their needs are: service, price, fear of failure, overstocking, etc.
(4) Explain how your product or idea will help them.
(5) Don't oversell: identify your best talents and promise only that.
(6) Don't cross the line and push for an order or approval on the first round. Offer to come back or allow voting members to study the proposal. Offer to meet with individuals at their convenience.
(7) Be persistent, even if you fail. The world won't come to an end, and tomorrow may make another effort more productive.
(8) Emphasize extraordinary value: Demonstrate your skill by giving clients or associates "more for their money."

I had a terrible time with everything I touched. This morning my collar button fell off. On my way to work. my briefcase handle fell off, and when I opened my office door, the handle fell off. I have to take a leak, but I'm afraid to go to the men's room. —**Larry Wilde**

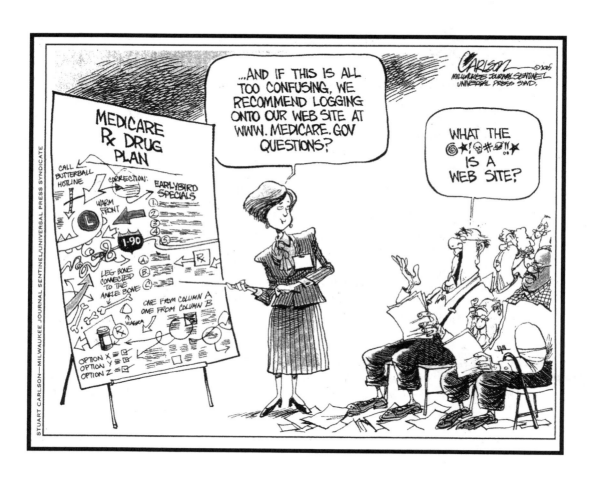

Trash Talk—Swearing and Cursing

*Some guy hit my fender, and I told him, "Be fruitful and multiply," but not in those words. —**Woody Allen***

A coping mechanism: Although the FCC is incensed by a virtual pandemic of verbal vulgarity in broadcast, and the general public often protests the crudity of blue comedy, the genie of profanity is out of the bottle and obscenity is universal, claims Natalie Angier in the *New York Times*. It is a natural outlet for rejection, anger and pain.

*When I say shit and motherfucker, people complain it's not proper. Well, I'd like to take them out to the parking lot and slam a car door on their fingers, and then they'll say shit and motherfucker. —**Redd Foxx***

Much ado about nothing: Researchers who study the evolution of language claim every language, dialect or patois, living or dead, has its share of forbidden speech. Blue-nosed English professors too often forget that Chaucer's *Canterbury Tales* were unabashedly bawdy and profane. Even the quintessential Bible abounds in naughty passages, and Shakespeare could hardly quill a stanza without inserting profanities of the day. Today the "f . . . word" is used so often, as an adjective or even as a full-bodied partner of the word "mother," that it has lost its power as an arousing epitaph. You know what the fuck I mean.

Wail to the chief: When former President George Herbert Walker Bush (the father, not the son or the Holy Ghost) gets down in the dumps, "I just swear at the TV set and yell at the bubblehead with whom I do not agree. I expect it is of no lasting benefit, but it sure feels good at the time." Cursing is often an amalgam of raw spontaneous feeling, and a curser rarely spews obscenities at random. Your reflexes react to the sound of such insults and all targets show signs of instant arousal. Obscenities can get under one's goose-bumped skin, and risqué interpolations are not easily forgotten. As a result, bad language can help wash away stress and anger and, in some settings, can be an effective means of venting aggression. It is a form of anger management that is often underappreciated, claims Timothy B. Jay, author of *Cursing in America*. There is even an illness, called coprolalia, a pathological and uncontrollable urge to curse.

Two children were looking at a bent nail. "What is it?" asked one. "I think it's called a god-dammit," said the other.

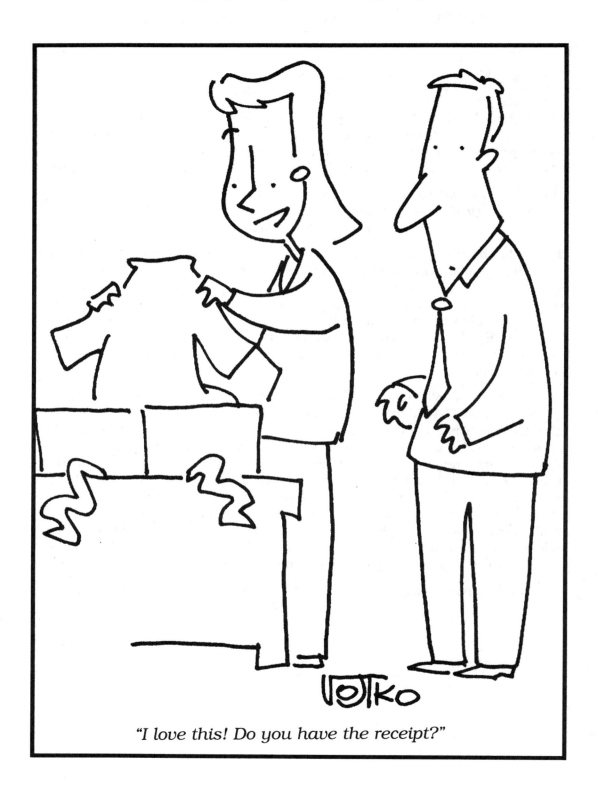

"I love this! Do you have the receipt?"

A Piece of the Rock—Going Shopping

We always hold hands. If I let go, she shops.

If you like going shopping, there are malls, department stores, restaurants, and Starbucks just down the street. If you hate shopping, then there's membership in The Church of Stop Shopping, a charade organization fathered by a fictional preacher called Reverend Billy. But for most, a diamond is not only forever, it's also the best revenge. If you can't afford diamonds, a new suit, a dress or a coat can brighten a bad day.

When women are depressed they either eat or go shopping. Men invade another country.
—Elayne Boosler

Oh Jackie! Jackie Kennedy loved clothes and the more sexual binges her husband had, the more shopping binges she would take for revenge. This fact may have been the inspiration for Neil Simon's line in his play *California Suite,* when a wife, who finds a call girl in her husband's hotel room, is asked "What are you going to do about it?" She answers, "I'm going out shopping to Rodeo Drive and I'm going to spend every cent you've got!" By the roar of audience approval, it's the play's most appreciated as well as oft-quoted line. And I can tell you I was sorry my wife saw the play.

I'm a shopaholic. I especially like to shop for shoes, because I don't have to take off my clothes. But if I do, I expect a much bigger discount. **—Bea Carroll**

A recent survey indicates that 15 percent of women who feel rejected turn to booze, 22 percent rely on caffeine, but 30 percent alleviate their stress by going shopping. They feel shopping reasserts their independence, that it challenges them with new things to conquer. And what a lovely trophy case!

My VISA card was stolen two months ago, but I don't want to report it. The guy who stole it is using it less than my wife. **—Johnny Carson**

When they're depressed, as scripted in the movie *In Her Shoes,* women most prefer to buy shoes—perhaps hoping they'll be going somewhere. Men, on the other hand, prefer sport shirts—perhaps daydreaming of a resort facility. Taking the time to shop carefully requires intense concentration, and figuring out how to pay for it requires even more.

I went shopping last week for feminine protection. I looked at all the products and decided on a .38 revolver. **—Karen Ripley**

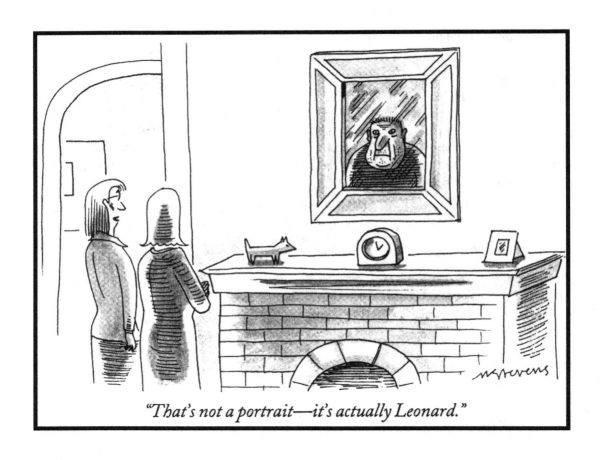

"That's not a portrait—it's actually Leonard."

Sin and Rescind—Getting Revenge

You can catch more flies with honey than with vinegar. But who wants flies?

Alex the grate: Revenge sounds better than it tastes. There is no such thing as "getting even" because there are no benchmarks at the start or the finish. And there is limited satisfaction. The rejection anger may be dissipated, but even if your revenge plan is successful, your disappointment will never disappear. When Nelson Mandela was asked if he could ever forgive his jailers, he said "When I walked out of the gate I knew that if I continued to hate these people I was still in prison."

I hate Father's Day. I can never find the right card because they are all too nice.
—Margaret Smith

Dumpster: Jill, a young lady in Michigan, was unceremoniously dumped by her long-time beau. "He used me, abused me, broke my heart, and threw me away. What was equally galling was that, despite my dire prediction that he would get hit by lightning, he became wildly successful. He fools everyone. They sing his praises and celebrate his glory. I want to scream and tell everyone the naked truth about him, and I know all about his being naked." But Carolyn Hax of the *Washington Post* claims that back-talking is the worst kind of revenge. It's also dangerous. "What you know," she warned, "does have its limits. He could have had an epiphany or a slow-motion maturing, even regret deeply the jerk he once was. But no matter how big a jerk he was, he's not your jerk anymore. What matters now—and always—is how well you're doing. Tend to your unhealed wounds. Then find your new post-heartbreak life, and live it."

My husband looked at Playboy and said, "How come you don't have any chest?" And I said, "When you married me, I didn't have a chest, and you didn't seem to care. But when I married you, you had a head full of hair." —Sue Costello

Sexual stimulant: Christina Aguilera uses her sex and make-up as protective armor. She feels vulnerable from men, paparazzi, and entertainment executives who think a woman who's assertive at work is a bitch. So Aguilera actually feels safest on stage dancing in a teeny bikini. Look, but don't touch. She feels it's important for women to share their story with other women who have been abused. When Aguilera was growing up, her father was emotionally and physically abusive to her and her mother. When her parents fought, she would run up to her room, put on a recording of *The Sound of Music* and sing out the window. Today, her hot, practically naked gyrations are not as intended to be provocative as they are to be statements of empowerment. By expressing herself sexually, Aguilera hopes to overcome her hatred of men who sexually abuse young women. "I am not a sexual tease," she pleads. "I think women are sensual, beautiful beings. Like music, sex can be an escape."

My ex-wife . . . what was her name again? Oh, yeah, plaintiff. —David Letterman

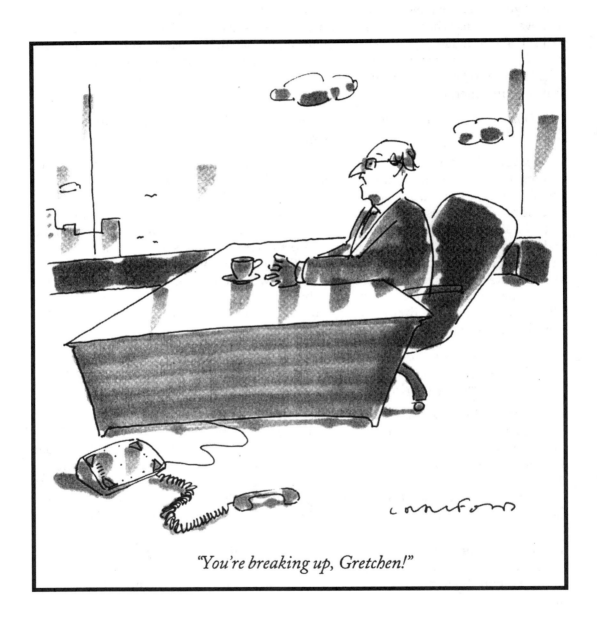

"*You're breaking up, Gretchen!*"

A Smashing Success—Getting It Off Your Chest and Onto the Floor

*They told me to ask for an office that was a stone's throw away from the boss, but then I found out that he had great aim. —**Mel Helitzer***

Air apparent: Outbursts that are out of proportion to the situation, like taking inexpensive pottery or a glass object and smashing it against the wall. As the pieces go flying, hopefully not in someone's eye, you can vent your anger in a way that's more legal than road rage, now called intermittent explosive disorder. John Kudlacet, who went into ceramic art because it was easier to sell than a painting, creates "rocking pots," which are perfect for throwing against the wall. "Otherwise," he said, "it's not functional at all." He knows the need for it because "as an artist, you've got to have an ego. You can't let rejection deter you."

How to end up Baroque: Michael Caine claims that he never loses his temper. "Instead, I go home and smash or rip out the windows." Someone asked, "Since you're a knight of the British Empire, were they stained glass windows?" "They were when I was finished with them," he answered.

A crashing success: Smashing something is a juvenile attempt to end anger immediately. You are generally not so eloquent to be able to hurl memorable insults. So by lashing out, throwing any object within reach, you are trying to wound or kill—even your mirror. Robert Ardrey, an anthropologist, believes our primate ancestors were carnivorous apes who made weapons that would destroy other animals when their territory was endangered. If they didn't have weapons, they threw rocks, and stoning other people to death is still a Middle East matinee.

Feat First: A survey claims that 40 percent of all women have hurled footwear at a man. They use satin bedroom slippers in coquettish pique, blue flats for mundane matters, spike-heeled pumps when they want to make a strong point and 50-pound hiking books when they're taking no prisoners. Anger can be harmful to your health if it's bottled up. The only bottle you should use has a liquor label on it.

Godfather One: It took Sofia Coppola a long time to find herself without needing her father, legendary movie director Francis Ford Coppola, at her side. She lived the life of a dilettante. She enrolled in art school, worked as a fashion designer's assistant and tried to be a photographer. When none of those worked, wrote Evgenia Peretz, her father cast her in *Godfather, Part III,* in a part that was universally panned. Then she tried directing her own films and hit bottom when her first was greeted with a magazine cover that proclaimed, "She ruined her father's film, now she's ruining one of her own." So she took Dad's photo and smashed it against the wall. "If you have a problem, you can't keep turning to your dad," she said. "You have to work harder just to prove you're not some spoiled girl." Since that smashing moment, she has become an accomplished director with such films as *The Virgin Suicides* and *Lost in Translation.*

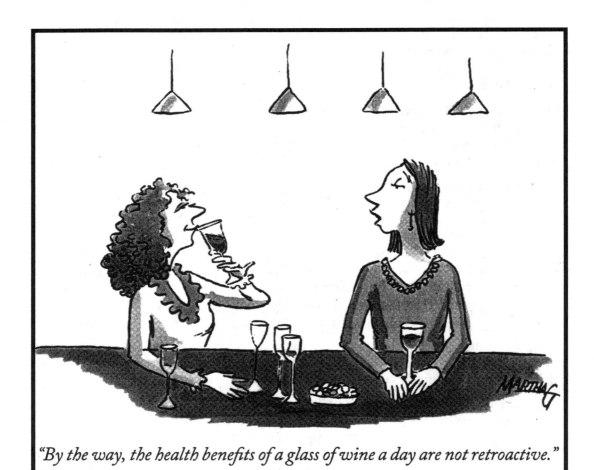

"By the way, the health benefits of a glass of wine a day are not retroactive."

Bottoms Up—Getting Drunk

They're putting warning labels on liquor "Caution! Alcohol can be dangerous to pregnant women." That's ironic. If it weren't for alcohol, most women would never be that way. **—Rita Rudner**

Men's room: While only 15 percent of women say that they turn to liquor when they're depressed, more than 65 percent of men grab for a shot as the second act of a major rejection. The first act is cursing.

The first purpose of alcohol is to make English your second language.
—Robin Williams

A stein's throw away: There are almost as many, but more appropriate, nicknames for an alcoholic drink as there are for a penis—a few of which are a belt, a shot, a nightcap, a pick-me-up, an eye-opener, and a hair of the dog. As a treatment for rejection, alcohol is a quick fix. It works in minutes—as do Valium and its cousins—and, despite the legal age limit, is more easily purchased and is less expensive.

I envy people who drink. At least they know what to blame everything on.
—Oscar Levant

Pour it on: It requires no discipline to use, although more books have been written on how to make a martini than on toilet training. But the dangers are also heavily advertised. Drinking responsibly is the mantra of all liquor advertising, and because it makes you fuzzy and uncoordinated, it produces gross cognitive and motor disabilities. In fact, motor concern is acute in more ways than one. Equally dangerously, it can cause deadly liver damage, brain damage and, as members of AA proselytize, it can become addictive.

Drinking makes such fools of people, and people are such fools to begin with, that it's compounding a felony. **—Robert Benchley**

I'll drink to that: Songwriter Chad Stuart claims the best recipe for rejection is a gin and tonic. The second best is a second gin and tonic. "While it works wonders," he said, "it's not that simple. The drinks have to be at the end of the day, and they have to be in a garden overlooking a fishpond, with the water bubbling over the rocks both inside and outside the glass. This scene continually reminds me that, no matter what the sadness, it's not the end of the world and that life goes on."

People who drink to drown their sorrow should be told that sorrow knows how to swim.
—Ann Landers

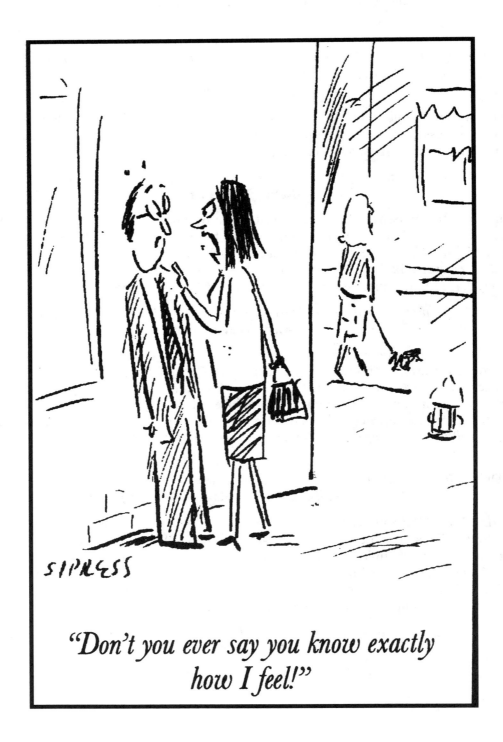

"Don't you ever say you know exactly how I feel!"

You Must Feel Awful—
Reflecting Their Feelings

It's no wonder that people are so horrible when they start life as children.
—Kingsley Amis

Now hear this: A parent should never scold a child that's been rejected, but empathize with them. In many ways, adults require the same amount of stroking as children do. They want sympathy and they want to be heard. It is fruitless to turn both requests down.

Why is it so easy to love our parents, and so hard to get them to love us? This is one of those questions that makes life so rich and psychiatrists richer.

Sects is a pity: More importantly, researchers have found that children as young as five who were chronically rejected by classmates were more likely to withdraw from school activities and scored lower on standardized tests. When a child doesn't do well at school, the teacher gets the blame: "She doesn't like me." The parent's incorrect answer would be, "I'm sure she wasn't upset without any reason. Teachers are so often overworked. Tell me exactly what you did wrong." At which point the child becomes even more incensed because the parent seems to be siding with the teacher. She feels misunderstood, one of the most painful emotions a child has.

Cry me a story: According to psychologist Alice Ginott the correct answer is "You must feel awful, Debbie. Let me give you a big hug. Then, let's talk about it and see what we can do together." This type of response is more effective because now the child feels important that you're giving her a chance to be heard sympathetically. This works for adults, too, and don't leave off the hug.

Tact is the art of telling someone to lose 30 pounds without ever using the word "fat."

One of life's ultimate rejections is the death of a spouse. Shirley Lord, former beauty editor of *Vogue*, wrote that during the three-day mourning period following the death of her husband, A. M. Rosenthal, former managing editor of the *New York Times*, she received condolence visits from hundreds of the most important people in the world. What she remembered vividly was that few of the mourners knew how to expresses their sympathies with meaningful remarks. "People don't know what to say," she wrote. "In fact, it would be better to say nothing at all—a hug, a squeeze on the shoulder, rather than 'My heart goes out to you.' I didn't want their heart, and I certainly didn't want them to say, 'I know how you feel.' And, while we were in agreement that he was a wonderful man and did so much for others, what I really wanted to hear, I admit it, was their recognition of how important I was in his life."

Dr. Edith Munger believes it is not as important to have answers for every problem as it is to get close to each other, to experience each other and to understand each other. Like believing in luck, for how else can we explain the success of those we don't like?

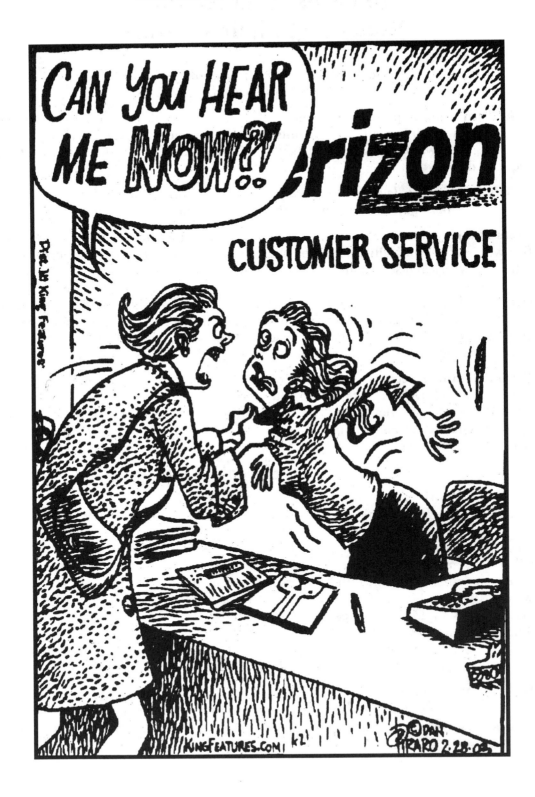

Listen, Damn It—Can You Hear Me Now?

To impact some people, all you have to do is listen. But there is nothing quite as annoying as having someone go on talking when you're interrupting. **—Bob Orben**

Honest Abe: Many times people bring you in to talk about their problems, and then they do all the talking and are grateful that all you did was listen. Historians have documented the oft-told story of Abraham Lincoln calling in an old friend to discuss one of the most important directives of his administration, the Emancipation Proclamation. Throughout the night, Lincoln talked non-stop, giving all his reasons and counter-arguments. When he was exhausted, he said good night and left without his friend having uttered an opinion.

If Lincoln were alive today, he'd roll over in his grave. **—President Gerald Ford**

A hushed secret: Avoid talking about yourself or turning the conversation to your own life. Don't say, "I know how you feel; the same thing happened to me," and then go into great detail about your own unhappy event. Listening right from the top of any discussion is a simple secret to making the relationship meaningful and yourself interesting. It means that you are in tune to someone else's feelings. The speaker's arm gestures, your empathetic nods and eye contact all show caring, reports Hap LeCrone of Cox News Service. "It's more effective than talking a lot and a lot easier to do. So listen to me."

Stress is when you wake up screaming and then you realize you haven't fallen asleep yet.

Zip your lip: Many so-called rejections are compliments that turn into unintentional harsh criticisms ("When you lose all that weight, you're going to be a beautiful young lady"). In business you can avoid a customer rupture by never interrupting a complaint until the speaker seems to be totally finished. Don't even ask questions unless it is totally necessary, because the tone of the question can often lead to additional vituperative answers. Instead immediately exhaust the sting of the complaint with positive recommendations, like agreeing to redo the project at no charge. Win the sale, not the argument.

In the middle of an asthma attack, my sister got an obscene phone call. After listening to her heavy breathing, the guy said, "Hey, did I call you or did you call me?"
—John Mendoza

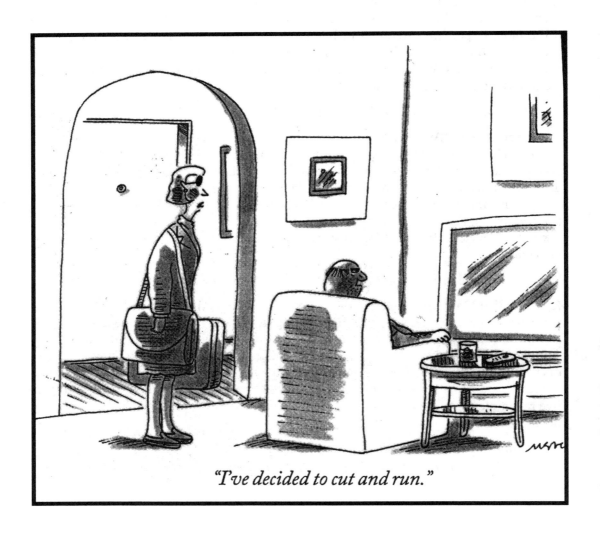

"I've decided to cut and run."

I Quit—Calling the Whole Thing Off

My husband and I celebrated our 38th wedding anniversary. And then I finally realized it. If I had killed the man the first time I thought about it, I'd have been out of jail by now.
—Anita Milner

Irrational: Orthodox conservatives point out that there are still twice as many marriages as divorces. The liberals, however, believe that the percentage of divorced couples would balloon if it weren't for self-serving family, financial, legal, or religious obstacles.

I will not cheat on my wife, because I love my house. **—Chas Elstner**

Legal eagles: Whatever your feelings, breaking off a relationship legally is increasingly popular as a rejection solution. Before women achieved financial independence, they often had to choose between love and money.

My mother always said, "Don't marry for money. Divorce for money."
—Wendy Liebman

In the new millennium, said the *Atlantic Monthly* editor Lori Gottlieb, the choice is now more often between love and offspring. According to the National Center for Health Statistics, the number of babies born to unmarried women rose by 290 percent from 1980 to 2002. Forecasting the future, there will be fewer religious weddings and more civil ceremonies. Also, the number of legal marriage contracts will slowly erode and be replaced by informal partnerships, defined by simple letters of agreement that can be terminated by either party without legal hassle.

I'm against gay marriage. I think marriage is a sacred Catholic union between a man and a pregnant woman. **—Craig Kilborn**

Slave trade: For males, this will mean trading a female slave contract for their freedom to roam the cattle range, and for females, they are giving up a legal security blanket for the right to create a new container for an independent, simpler, more creative and less angry life.

Baby, don't leave me: The groups that may suffer the most are children whose fears of abandonment will start sooner after infancy and last until maturity, although the category of parents who typically report the most parenting satisfaction—who feel they're doing the best job—is divorced dads.

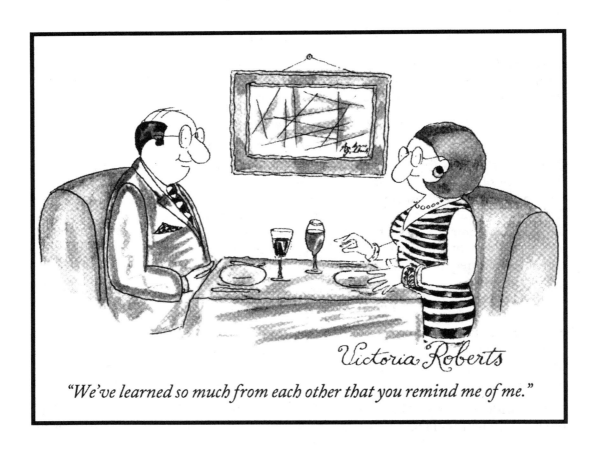

"We've learned so much from each other that you remind me of me."

The Magic Touch—Getting a Mentor

Hard is not hopeless: The world is too complex and life styles are too hectic for rugged individualism. Everyone needs a support system, so get a mentor, a coach, a teacher, or a respected friend who can be effective in support, in experience, and in giving a needed push. Ask the person to be positive, but truthful. You cannot ever know too much. Martha Stewart claims her mentors were experts at what they knew—a gardener at some estate, a farmer who milks his own cows, a professor, or some authors she admired. "I've informally constructed mentors in this structure in my life," she said.

Life is a series of problems: A mentor is a trusted, knowledgeable, experienced individual with a vested interest in your accomplishing more. Mentors are readily available. For business owners, such professional associations as Young Presidents' Organization (YPO), Young Entrepreneurs' Organization (YEO), The Executive Committee and the National Association of Women Business Owners (NAWBO) provide seminars and guidance material. Most universities have innovative industrial incubators that include support from the school's best research instructors. In addition, most industry associations can recommend the names of seasoned retired members who can counsel neophytes.

The thing about being a professor is that if you can just make one student successful, if you can just make one student see the light, if you can just make one student ready for the outside world, then you're still stuck with nineteen failures. **—Mel Helitzer**

All you need to no! The counseling world is also filled with charlatans because it is a multi-billion-dollar business. There is an army of uncertified, self-appointed contemporary snake oil salesmen who can tell you in a five-minute broadcast, or a 200-word news column or a 300-page book how to instantly solve every personal problem, from how to have faith in your own instincts to whether you should leave your spouse and children for a better world. There are hundreds of hyperbolic self-help book titles such as *How to Make the Rest of Your Life the Best of Your Life* (Mark Victor Hanson), *All I Really Need to Know I Learned in Kindergarten* (Robert Fulghum), *The Seven Spiritual Laws of Success* (Deepak Chopra), *10 Stupid Things Women Do to Mess Up Their Lives* (Laura Schlessinger), and *Healing the Soul of America* (Marianne Williamson) that equalize instant therapy and instant coffee. In his book *SHAM,* an acronym for the Self-Help and Actualization Movement, Steve Salerno offers a mind-boggling expose of an industry that is causing real damage to its paying (and paying again) customers.

Q & A: Wouldn't this book, too, fall into the SHAM category? The difference is that this book's readers have 101 personal options for ameliorating a rejection rather than be subjected to an unconditional psychological facsimile of The Ten Commitments.

Since you have to make choices every day, the first choice is to decide who you are.

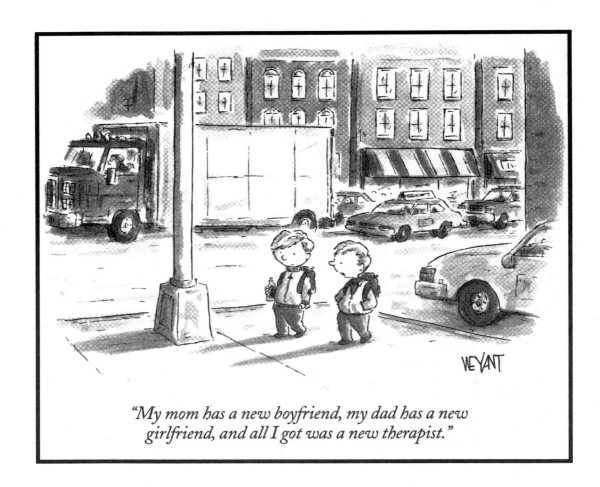

"*My mom has a new boyfriend, my dad has a new girlfriend, and all I got was a new therapist.*"

The Mouth That Roared—Going Into Analysis

The aim of psychoanalysis is to relieve people of their neurotic unhappiness so that they can become normally unhappy. —Sigmund Freud

Artificial happiness: Today's erudites believe therapy and drugs are the entitlement to the happiness that was in Jefferson's mind when he penned "the pursuit of happiness." Whether they are required or not, such drugs as Zoloft, Wellbutrin, Prozac, and a medicine chest of other antidepressants are now the rage as prescriptions for artificial happiness. A study claims that people diagnosed with a major depression start to change for the better as soon as the doctor writes a prescription. Even insurance companies are big supporters, preferring to pay for pills instead of hours of costly psychiatric counseling.

After 12 years of therapy, my psychologist said three words that brought tears to my eyes. He said, "No hablo ingles." —Ronnie Shakes

Splenda an hour with me: But drugs are only temporary mental band-aids, according to many psychiatrists who see it as their duty to eradicate ordinary unhappiness completely. Anti-depressant medication has gone up 50 percent in the last five years, but group therapy or personal counseling sessions are more long-term.

I don't consider myself to be an analyst's patient but a sustaining member of his financial supporters. —Mel Helitzer

They counsel that rejection can be the forerunner of jarring depression. Here are several of the personality changes that signal trouble:

(1) A social withdrawal and loss of interest in daily life.

(2) A major shift in behavior, such as long crying spells, trouble sleeping, decreased appetite, or changes in energy level.

(3) Despondency that lasts for a more than couple of weeks.

(4) Difficulty adjusting to a new responsibility, like new parenting.

(5) Refusal to confide in family or friends.

(6) Self-mutilation, such as major skin cuts due to substance abuse.

*Neurotics build castles in the air, psychotics live in them. My mother cleans them.
—Rita Rudner*

Now and Zen: Don't look at the downside when it's time to call for help. Don't hesitate to enter therapy because you'll think you'll discover dark and embarrassing secrets deep inside you. If these thoughts do exist, it's also the time to turn on the light. Remember, even if it's 98 percent the other person's fault, it's still 2 percent your fault. Professional therapy can free you from this excess baggage.

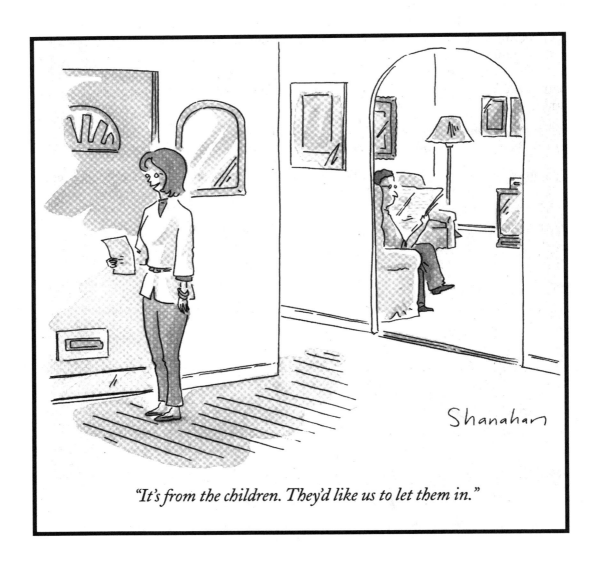

"It's from the children. They'd like us to let them in."

Just What the Bible Says—Forgive and Forget

Forgive your enemies. Nothing annoys them so much. —**Oscar Wilde**

Emotional boomerang: It's difficult to give away kindness. It keeps coming back to you. Avoid an emotional wheelchair that keeps you from making peace with the past. Start with small courtesy offerings, ignore little pricks of rejection, and then grow to events that make a dramatic impact.

I first learned about rejection as a kid when my yo-yo never came back.
—**Rodney Dangerfield**

This, too, shall pass: Remember that most rejections are temporary. It's better if you nudge yourself in a helpful direction. If it won't matter a year from now, why should it matter today? One of the most popular books in recent years is Richard Carlson's *Don't Sweat the Small Stuff.* "Our time is precious," preaches Carlson. "The best antidote for pain is joy. Learn to let go."

If you find yourself in a hole, the first thing to do is stop digging.

Time and time again: You can get as addicted to being rejected as you can with any other strong emotion or chemical product. Evidence of this addiction is the frequency you rerun past rejections through your mental projector like an all-time classic movie. Negative feelings become habitual by taking every negative incident personally. Some believe displaying perpetual anger makes them powerful. Others believe confessions like "It was all my fault" will make them sympathetic. As a self-anointed martyr, they nurse the pain for years. Both beliefs are wrong. In truth, most rejections have little to do with us. It is more likely that the event that rejected you was not properly organized, or the other person had a personal problem of which you were unaware, or, the most unflattering, you just weren't that important in the immediate scheme of things.

Someone said to me, "Make yourself a sandwich." Well, if I could make myself something, it wouldn't be a sandwich. I'd make myself a horny 18-year-old billionaire.
—**George Carlin**

Keystone cope: One of the best possible keys to healing this type of insecurity is the act of forgiveness. Take a deep breath, get rid of your anger, and quit thinking you're the victim. A forgiving attitude doesn't require you to deny your pain or heal a relationship. Even if you have to talk to a chair, forgiveness is a gift to yourself. Faster than two Tylenols, you can reduce stress and feel better immediately. "If you don't expect perfection in others, you can develop a new mind-set by eliminating self-blaming statements," according to Judy Tatelbaum, author of *You Don't Have to Suffer.*

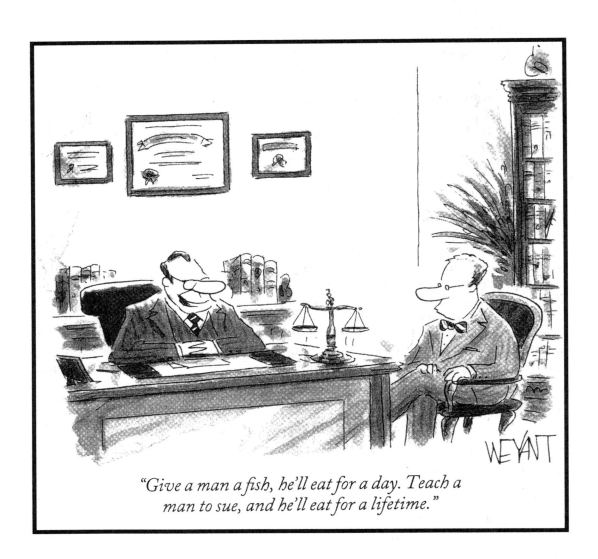

"Give a man a fish, he'll eat for a day. Teach a man to sue, and he'll eat for a lifetime."

A Labor of Love—Being a Teacher

You know, professor, your class makes me think. Like what in the hell am I doing here?
—Mel Helitzer student

Hey, coach: It sounds paradoxical, but when you're feeling rejected, one antidote is to cast away your own problems by counseling other people. Parents do it daily. Therapists often decided to get into psychiatry after they spent long stretches in analysis. By offering to be another's coach, you need to help them set goals. Ask them to analyze the way they are unique, putting on the table their positive personalities and objectives. Then listen to yourself as you hand out advice to others. You'll not only reinforce the knowledge that everyone has rejection problems, and that not only aren't theirs as bad as they first imagined, but that facing up to them is the first step toward avoiding problems in your own future.

If it's working, keep doing it. If it's not working, stop doing it. If you don't know what to do, don't do anything. **—Melvin Konner**

Teacher's pet peeve: As a teacher, you work with groups of students. But a major danger lies in a public reprimand, a taboo in the work place. Criticizing one student's work in a classroom setting can be humiliating but necessary in order to train the group. This is the time for subtle remarks, such as, "Your proposal may not be the most logical. Here is another possibility. What do you think?"

Love is to care about other people. Charm is the ability to make other people believe you're truly interested in them.

You can write! When Erma Bombeck enrolled at Ohio University as a freshman in 1946, she wanted to be a writer. But her English professor kept degrading her essays, and she couldn't get a job at the daily student newspaper. After two years, she transferred to the University of Dayton, still floundering over what her major might be. One of her new communication instructors, a Jesuit brother, wrote on one of her submissions, "Erma, you can *write*!" Delighted with the encouragement, Erma switched into journalism, got a job as a cub reporter for the *Dayton Daily News,* and eventually blossomed into one of the country's most talented and beloved humor columnists. When she died, her estate left Dayton University all her papers and a sizeable donation so that the university could conduct an annual writer's conference under the title, "You can write!" As a journalism professor at Ohio University, I was invited to give a keynote speech at the first Bombeck conference in 2000, and then I understood why I was invited. So I could return to OU, meet with the faculty of the English department and kick ass.

The best way to make a long story short is to forget the punch line.

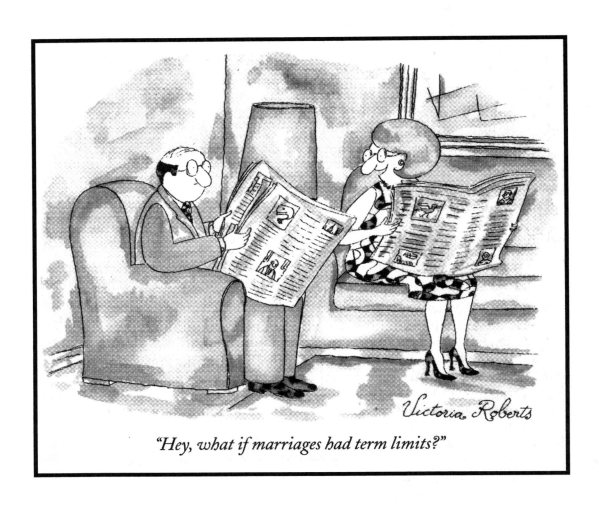

"Hey, what if marriages had term limits?"

Last Rights—Eliminating Disparagement

*Sophisticated people have retirement plans. Rednecks, on the other hand, play the lottery. Our plan is that when we hit the Pick Six, we're going to add a room onto our trailer so we don't have to sleep with Grandpa no more. —**Jeff Foxworthy***

Anger is a normal human emotion. It is like the flaring of a match, a sudden searing flame with a short life, or as steam from a boiling teapot. The best way to vent it is to turn off the flame.

When you're angry, it's difficult to learn. A clenched fist can not accept a gift.
—John Roger McWilliams

Daily express: Anger can be expressed by words and pitching, but true violence is unconstructive. So is plunging into alcohol or drug-related products such as tobacco or depressants. Instead, get physical in healthy ways. It's more practical to slap a cold washcloth on your face, take deep breaths, take a long walk, talk to an empty chair, smash a tennis ball, but leave your poor dog alone. Martin Luther, in the 16th century, believed that "manual labor—like harnessing the horse or spreading manure—was a good way to get rid of fear," reports Pastor Lynn Miller. Write a vituperative letter but trash it before you're tempted to send it. Instead, give your adversaries the silent treatment, known as the cold shoulder.

I wish men would get more in touch with their feminine side and become self-destructive.
—Betsy Salkind

Toss 'em: Remove the following words from your daily vocabulary: *rejection, shame, anxiety, fear, embarrassment, and disgust.* If you don't constantly recoil from them, you won't be controlled by them.

Runaway disagreements: Conflicts snowball when you get into a crazy cycle of reacting to casual things other people say in an attempt to trivialize a negative question. Suppose a wife whines, "This is the worst meal I've ever made," and the husband retorts, "No, it's not, honey," the wife may react negatively, "Are you saying that I've made thousands of worse meals?" Or when one spouse wakes up feeling fat and ugly and the other suggests a book on diet control, chaos can ensue. The magic bullet solution for this error, claims Emerson Eggerich in his book *Love and Respect,* is to immediately say, "I'm sorry. I didn't mean to hurt you."

Stop and retrench: Many squabbles are rooted in the fact that one person did not understand the emotional needs of the other. It's just that women have a tendency to go on and on about the same subject, while men have a tendency to rush to a solution. According to John Gray, in his book *The Mars of Venus Diet and Exercise Solution,* it's much better to call a timeout and say, "I'd like to think about what you're saying, and then let's talk again."

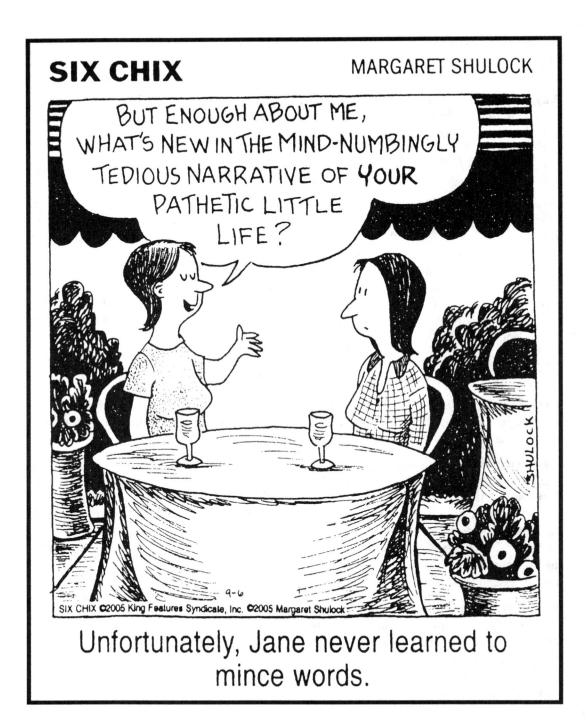

A League of Their Own—Associating With Positive People

Mother's Day card: *"Mom, you're the greatest. At least that's what all the guys at the construction site say."*

The power of positive people: Barbra Streisand's signature song "People," contains the line, "People, people who need people, are the luckiest people in the world." The benefit of a support group is arguably the most effective rejection strategy of them all. No one person develops anything completely on her own. Those who think they can live life alone are locked up in a prison of their own making. Bill Clinton claims that, to be secure, it's important that you like being around people who know more about any subject than you do. "In the end," he said, "you hear them out and then you can trust your own judgment."

Close to the edge: When Elizabeth was 25, she was devastated over a breakup with her fiancé. Her interest in her job went crashing. She starting eating everything on the table and her weight shot up. Her daily beverage went from beer to hard liquor—and lots of it. One night she was tossed out of a bar by the bouncer. Depressed, she isolated herself from everything and everyone in her life. She locked herself in her room and started to write a suicide note, but she was interrupted when a friend barged into her room. The friend called two other friends and they insisted that Elizabeth move in with them. Each took on a specific assignment. One channeled her eating habits to health foods, and within two weeks her weight started falling into place. Another accompanied Elizabeth to exercise classes and on shopping trips to help improve her appearance. As her figure, improved so did the attention she received from young men. The third friend encouraged her to join activity clubs and helped her to meet new people. The dedication and interest of her friends restored Elisabeth's belief in herself. "I will never forget it," she said. "I learned the support of friendship and the power of love."

Keep only cheerful friends. The grouches pull you down. **—George Carlin**

Hide and seek: How do you find positive people? Easy. Just stay away from negative people. Then visualize yourself as a celebrated champion so famous and successful that criticism bounces off your gold medals. Or you can look for a tragedy whose heroes to emulate. One such support group is Kate's Club, a grass roots club in Atlanta where a hundred kids who have lost a parent or a sibling can get camaraderie, support, and warmth from other kids who share similar sorrows. "It's nice to see," said founder Kate Atwood, "that even though your mom died prematurely, you can still turn out O.K." Sharon Blynn was in cancer remission for three years. It was a long and difficult struggle, so she helped found Bald is Beautiful, an organization that helps cancer patients feel beautiful while they fight for their lives. Actress Kate Hudson says that she protects herself from negative people in Hollywood by spraying herself with water crystals. "I carry some water with me all the time. When I'm around people with bad energy, I just put it on myself. It's not like holy water—just something to cleanse myself if someone's really negative."

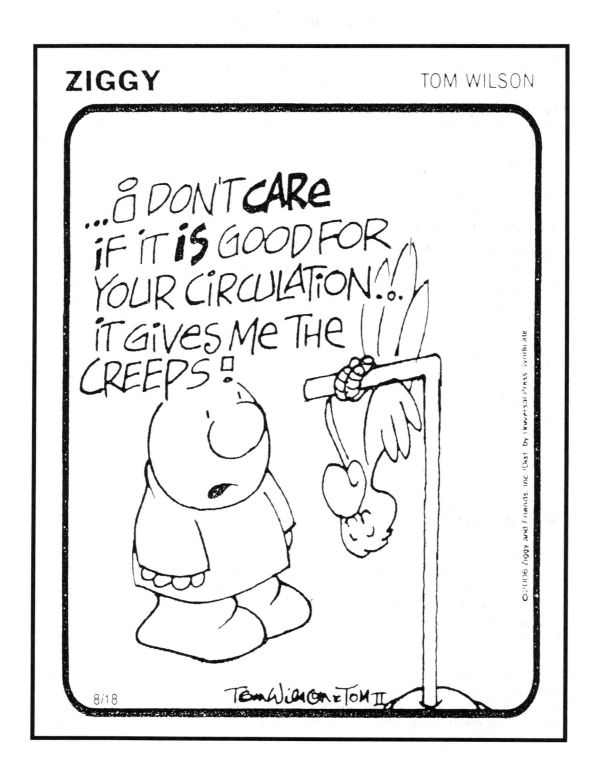

Guided Muscles—Working It Out

The first time I see a jogger smiling, I'll consider it. —**Joan Rivers**

The ball is just a metaphor: There is a correlation between exercise and a reduction in depression. It's never too late to get moving. Combining physical activity, from strolls to rock-climbing, with talk therapy sessions has become the latest rejection therapeutic rage—but it's actually been known for more than a century. In his book, *Conquering Anxiety and Depression Through Exercise,* Keith Johnsgard points out that, in the 1800s, Sigmund Freud walked his patients through the streets of Vienna or took a few along on vacations so they could garden, chop wood or stroll with the doctor. Today, public health experts recommend adults get thirty minutes of physical activity seven days a week. You don't have to run on a treadmill or play tennis. Just walk more, like taking the stairs instead of an elevator, and do more physical chores around the house.

If it weren't for the fact that the TV set and the refrigerator are so far apart, some of us wouldn't get any exercise at all. —**Joey Adams**

Get the stress out: The five basic rules for eliminating stress by physical activity are (1) breathe deeply and restore your oxygen supply, (2) get your rest, because a lack of sleep contributes to your feeling overwhelmed and irritable, (3) prioritize your day and start practicing time -management skills such as keeping a list and ranking them by value, (4) eliminate distractions, like telephone calls, voice mail, email, and unscheduled meetings so you can focus on the top of your priority list, and (5) make time to exercise every day. Your body as well as your mind needs time to recharge.

My grandmother began walking five miles a day when she was 82. Now, we don't know where the hell she is. —**Ellen DeGeneres**

Are hamsters laughing at us? Author Tony Schwartz claims you can seize more control of your life by understanding that human beings are complex energy systems that not only rhythmically expand and recover but also require a variety of energy systems in order to fire on all cylinders. A body workout is like peeling an onion. You unwind more and more with each layer. You feel lighter. Two of the most important energy sources are diet—not only what we eat, but how much and when we eat—and exercise. Without the right fuel in our tank, we tend to under perform. When we exercise right, we can get rewired. Schedule workouts with a friend or a trainer. That way, you'll be less likely to skip your sessions.

I am pushing 60. That's enough exercise for me. —**Mark Twain**

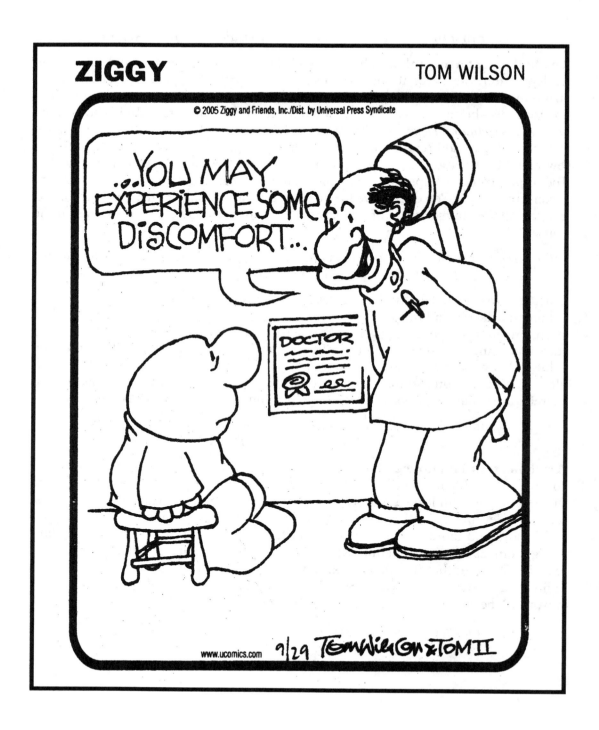

To Rite the Wrong—Nursing Your Wounds

*People say, "Don't watch your money. Watch your health." So one day I was at the club watching my health, and my ex-wife stole all my money. —**Jackie Mason***

Think positive: Experts debate how much isolation is healthy when you've been mentally wounded and just want to meditate. "Keep a list of happy reminiscences," says Jefferson A. Singer, "and whenever you feel sad, focus on one." Barbara Moe in her book *Coping with Rejection* agrees. Her favorite remedies are (1) choosing a special treat for yourself, (2) doing something nice for your body, (3) posting a motivating quote on your refrigerator door, and (4) reviewing, in a fan mail folder, complimentary letters and awards. Skim them on dark days. Your light will be better when you finish.

Dear diary, you won't believe this one. One of the best rejection antidotes, however, is to write nice things about yourself in a private journal or diary, choose what facts and captions for photos to include and what to leave out, what to exaggerate and what to justify. Do it for relief not for publication. "Write is right," says singer Christina Aguilera. "It's the best way for me to eradicate anger and chaos."

Blamestutorial: Anderson Cooper was born in a family of fame and wealth—his mother was heiress Gloria Vanderbilt. But tragedy struck twice—when he was just ten, his father died during heart surgery. Ten years later, his brother committed suicide by jumping from a fourteen-story window. "How could they have left me to deal with their mess?" he wondered. As a CNN correspondent, Cooper has made a career of tracking grief around the world. "I wanted to be someplace where the pain outside matched the pain I was feeling inside." He purposely goes to dangerous places where pain is the most common horror. "I wanted to know why some survived and some didn't." To come to terms with his own family tragedies, he worked nonstop for over a year on a book. "An assumption one can not make is that grief ever ends," said author Kenneth Doka. "Once you have written it out, bad days are fewer and farther between."

*This guy I was dating was a dog. He'd keep sniffing around, scratching all over and was constantly looking for a place to bury his bone. —**Pamela Yager***

Carrying on the legacy: Terri Irwin plans to raise her kids to be as fearless as their famous father, Steve "The Crocodile Hunter," who was killed by a stingray barb. Because his show *Wild Animals* is still on TV every morning, his pre-school children think their father is just on his next adventure. "We are still a family," says Terri. "I talk to Steve out loud. I write him letters. It's quite therapeutic. He showed me not to panic about every little thing. To keep my spirit alive, I tell my children that there are different kinds of strength. I'm teaching them to tie knots."

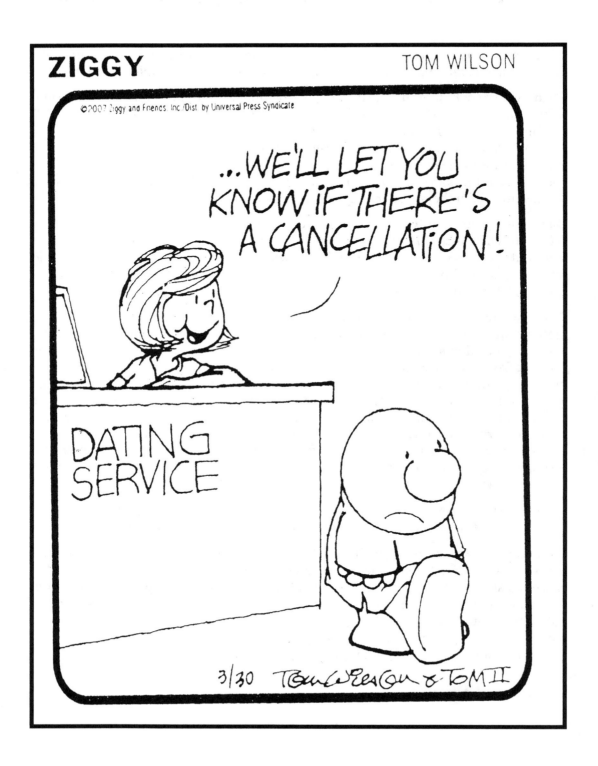

One More Time—Being Persistent

*"I just kept going up there and swinging at 'em." —**Babe Ruth***

The word for tomorrow: Elaine Savage believes that the opposite of rejection is perseverance. Avoid negative thinking. Compare success to infinity. You know it's there even if you never see it. Like a champion racehorse, your best odds for success are to put on blinders of discipline. Common sense does not guarantee success, which is why there are so many overweight people and so much communicable disease from unprotected sex.

Who am I? How did I come into this crazy world? Why was I not consulted?
*—**Soren Kierkegaard***

Perpetual motion: Do not give way, do not give in, and do not give up. Examples: Katie Couric wanted to be a news anchor when only men were being hired as announcers, and Ruth Bader Ginsburg, now a Supreme Court justice, graduated at the top of her class at Harvard Law School but couldn't get a job at any New York law firm because they had never before hired a woman. Sir Edmund Hilary failed several times to climb Mount Everest before he finally succeeded. As you grow older, you accumulate knowledge like a rolling snowball. You just aren't the age you are. You're all the ages you have ever been, wrote Kenneth Koch.

*Life is not measured by the number of breaths, we take but by the moments that take your breath away. That's why it's more important to tell people whom you love that you love them at every opportunity. —**George Carlin***

The eleventh-hour hello: Marcia Cross may be one of the *Desperate Housewives* on TV, but she was a desperate single at 40 in real life. She had had a five-year relationship with an actor 24 years her senior—perhaps, she admits, it was a father-daughter thing—but then he suddenly developed a brain tumor. "He died in my bed!" reported Cross, "and all I had left was the pride that I had taken care of him and given him a good death." She got a part in the hot TV show, but her social life was several degrees below zero. She tried dating services, quickly despaired of pressure-filled blind dates, and found herself all alone for the Christmas holidays. "What happened then was crazy," she admits. She followed a handsome stranger into a flower shop, gave him her number, and didn't even introduce herself. A few days later, he called for a date but she had to turn him down. He still didn't know who she was. "That's the night I am being nominated for a Golden Globe Award," she told him. "You know what a Globe is?" "Of course," he said, "but I didn't know you can win an award for changing a light bulb." With that kind of humor, he got a date and only weeks later he got a bride. "That's not the way to do it," Cross advises, "but taking a chance can produce an incredible sense of gratefulness."

I was married for two years, a long time if you count it by all those ten-minute segments.
*—**Charisse Savarin***

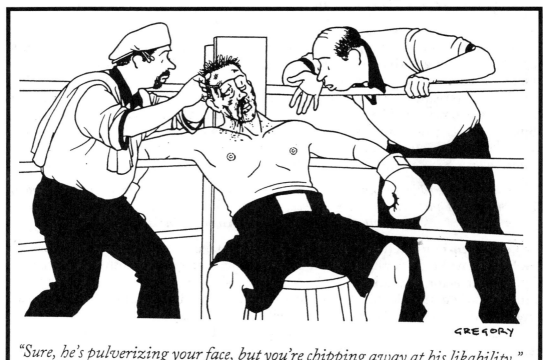

"Sure, he's pulverizing your face, but you're chipping away at his likability."

All For One—Seeing the Big Picture

Endure, grieve, cry, but move on. The only person with us for our entire life is ourself.
—George Carlin

The big picture: A consistent .300 hitter in major league baseball soon becomes a millionaire, even though he technically was out seven out of ten times. Actors in a Broadway smash hit have good and bad shows even if they've performed the part 1,000 times (which is why Hollywood films shoot the same scene multiple times). Being despondent every time one thing goes wrong is buying a one-way ticket to the psychiatric ward.

I sold my house this week. I got a good price for it, but it made my landlord mad as hell.
—Garry Shandling

Critics are often wrong: A. O. Scott, of the *New York Times,* admits that creative art critics are often out of touch with the ever-changing market. He and most other major film reviewers yelled "bomb" in rejecting both *Pirates of the Caribbean* and *The DaVinci Code.* But within weeks, the pirate film became the world's biggest blockbuster, earning over $500 million, and the DaVinci drama pocketed the biggest opening weekend gross in the history of Sony. "These are just two examples of the discrepancies between what critics think and how the public behaves," he wrote. "The more vexing issue is what, exactly, critics are for." They are darned if their breathless praise is too positive and damned if they complained too wildly. The moral is not to let even professional judges narrow your focus or impair your decision-making process. Evaluating the true impact of your rejection on your daily life will help you shake it off faster and avoid erratic mental clarity.

The trouble with doing something right the first time is that nobody appreciates how difficult it was.

Tiny tears: For example, is it necessary to control your grief? Crying or cursing, for example, are natural reactions to rejection. They both act as a release. And cursing God, while frowned upon by religious zealots, is so automatic that it occurs faster than stamping your feet. While it may take a conscious physical effort to avoid complaining and smashing objects, you can rechannel your physical displays through organized athletic activities, fitness programs in the gym, and even with Chinese balls at home.

Grow up: The actor Alicia Silverstone has been starring in films since she was 14 and, incredibly, living by herself at 15. "I think of all the mistakes I made feeling pseudo-sophisticated. I thought I was on fire. Now the only thing I want is to be a big sister to that little girl, and go take care of her because she didn't know how much she was lacking in that loving, supportive way. Like, I'm a vegan activist, so I changed my diet and I started to feel a million times better. My body started to look better. My skin started to look better. My nails got really strong. I learned to take care of my own body, and it changed me as a woman."

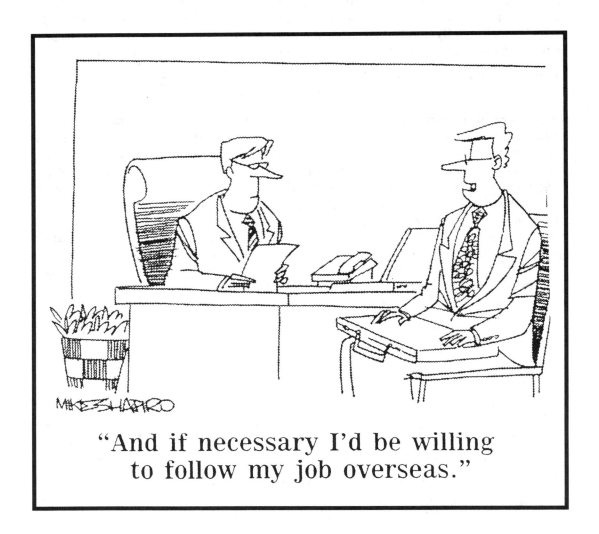

"And if necessary I'd be willing to follow my job overseas."

Repackaged—Being Versatile

Whatever goes up must come down, but don't expect it to come down where you can find it. **—Lily Tomlin**

If you insist upon being rigid, you may be dead. People get into ruts. They're fearful of making a change. You can't always just go with the flow. You have to be versatile. "When you're through changing," warns Martha Stewart, "you're through!" Apply your ability to the opportunities of the moment.

My grandmother was a very tough woman. She buried three husbands. Two of them were only napping. **—Rita Rudner**

The bag lady: Food Network chef Paula Deen's panic attacks started the morning the hospital notified her that her father had died in an auto accident. "When you're a teenager and something snatches away the rug you call security," she said, "you land on your ass." Then she rationalized that God had taken her father as a sign she, too, was going to die soon. Her acrophobia kept her fearful of leaving her house. Sometimes she couldn't breathe or stop trembling. Her salvation was cooking and packing lunch baskets for local office workers, and that led her to her own restaurant, now one of the most famous in Savannah. "I'm a true steel magnolia," she claims, "because southern women have unfailing survival instincts. Cooking saved my life."

A lot of people are afraid of heights. Not me. I'm afraid of widths. **—Steven Wright**

Come fly with me. Jennifer had only a few days to consider her dilemma. Her husband was being transferred by his Fortune 500 company to a medium-sized city in the Midwest. Even though it meant giving up her job as a top-flight public relations executive in New York, Jennifer went with him. After a few weeks organizing her new home and her children's schooling, she was eager to go back to work, but her new city didn't have a single PR firm, only a few one-man practitioners. She was frustrated that all her professional skills and the income they produced were going to waste.

Event planning: Jennifer prepared a few dummy profiles of local businessmen who each had an interesting story to tell and suggested them as samples of a free weekly column she would write for the local daily newspaper. The editor was delighted, especially with the word "free." The column was an opportunity for Jennifer to meet the top business leaders in the city several times—first when she arranged the meeting, secondly when she interviewed and photographed the subject, thirdly when she submitted the draft manuscript for approval, and finally after the article appeared, when she personally delivered a laminated copy of the printed story plus prints of all the photographs she took. During these meetings she subtly told them of her metropolitan experience as an event planner and offered to provide that service when they had need. Even small firms have business events such as sales meetings, trade shows, retirement roasts, and holiday celebrations that require organization, and within a year, Jennifer had an event assignment almost every week from fifteen clients.

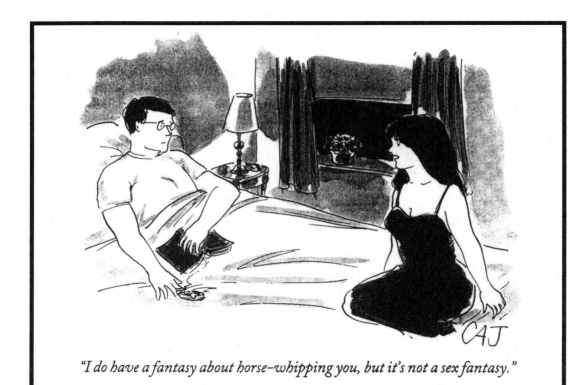

"I do have a fantasy about horse-whipping you, but it's not a sex fantasy."

Kneading the Best—Getting a Massage

*For my husband's last birthday, I booked a masseuse to come to the house. When I went to the door, there was an 18-year-old gorgeous blonde, who said, "I'm here to give your husband a massage." I said, "He's dead." —**Rita Rudner***

Stress it out: When someone touches your body, there is generally a chemistry charge that can be very positive. Tactile relationships have long been one of the most powerful elements of communication for establishing personal relationships, the main question being how reciprocal are the feelings of the other party. Giving a massage to others is also a valuable human contact. Consider getting a massage several times a week for maximum effect or at least once a week for a month. Use scented oils, dimmed lights and music and, as the masseuse works, let your mind wander uncensored through the journey.

Spotting relief: The four most popular massage techniques are (1) the Swedish massage, that increases circulation with long strokes, kneading motions or friction, but unfortunately a beautiful, blonde Swedish masseuse is rarely available, (2) the trigger-point massage, sometimes known as the "ouch" massage, that uses fingertip pressure to reduce sensitivity in a muscle, (3) the deep-tissue massage that is done with kneading and long strokes that aim at deeper muscle layers to help with chronic muscle pain, and (4) the hot-stone massage, that uses heated volcanic basalt placed on your back that helps loosen muscles when massaged with the stones. There is another popular massage, but that stimulant may not be legal in some areas.

*I'm 100 percent Sicilian. Not all Sicilians are in the mob. Some are in the witness protection program. —**Tammy Pescatelli***

Take a bite out of a small bit: Take on an immediate obligation or project, and reward yourself often, even once a day, with every successful part-time accomplishment. The rewards need not be prestigious. For children, and many adults, a hug from a member of the family may be a memorable reward.

*I stayed at a hotel that advertised "We treat you like family." They were right. At nine o'clock in the morning, someone was banging on my door shouting, "When the hell are you gonna get a place of your own?" —**Brian McKim***

Short-term goals: Self-esteem improves with any positive reinforcement, so being goal oriented, even in a short-term project, is a catalyst for long-term confidence. Your self-assurance engine needs to be constantly refueled, and you can do this by keeping busy with small projects.

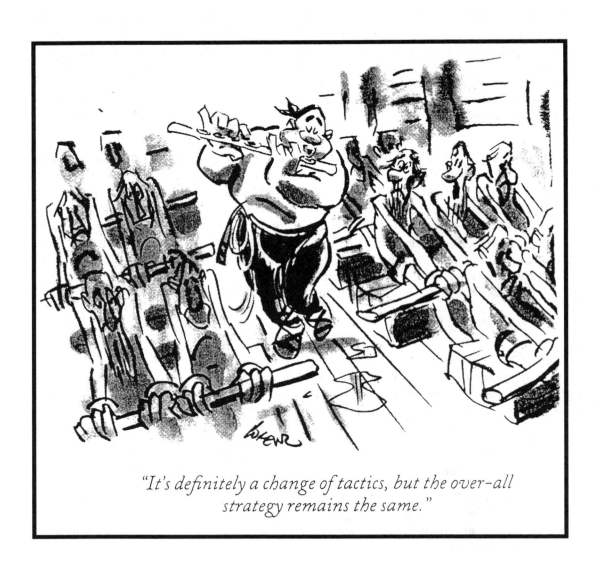

"It's definitely a change of tactics, but the over-all strategy remains the same."

Up Yours!—Finding an Alternative Goal

Two roads diverged in a wood, and I took the road less traveled by—State Troopers.

Redirect focus: The knee-jerk reaction to every rejection is to take things personally—that the criticism was directed solely at you. By assuming that every slight, physical or verbal, is directed at you, you are enhancing a conceit that is often incorrect. General negative remarks that are ethnic or physical in nature, laughter that appears to be smirking, criticism that is overheard but you assume is pinpointed at you, or sudden actions by an individual that seem impolite or disconcerting can be overreacted upon and cause a rush to bad judgment.

*"Bad judgment" has replaced "bad behavior." Now, when caught red-handed, public officials confess only to exercising "bad judgment," often accompanied by "mistakes were made." —**Jon Winokur***

Rejection can't kill you, but why take a chance? Start rebuilding your confidence with short-term successes, such as alternating simple and complex projects. As your batting average improves, you'll find the proper balance of easy and hard assignments.

*Blind people are complaining that seeing-eye dogs are expensive, difficult to train and hard to get. So I say, let's use midgets. They can use the work. —**Chris Rock***

God help us: A seminary student was upset that one of the pastors on the judging committee for her final exam suddenly got up in the midst of her demonstration sermon, walked out of the room and only returned when she had finished. This bothered her so much that she demanded an explanation from the senior pastor, only to find out that he had a prostrate problem, needed immediate relief, and decided not to come back into the room and disrupt her sermon a second time. This was a case of reverse egocentrism. In interpreting every slight, don't be so self-indulgent that you take it personally. You may not be that important.

*I think Kathy Griffin should get to know someone, and even be in love with them, before using them to degrade. —**Steve Martin***

Ready, aim, fire: Creative people, particularly, feel it is necessary to keep changing their target in life. Ridley Scott, a film director, said, "Changing your target keeps you insecure. And a little bit of insecurity is good for everyone."

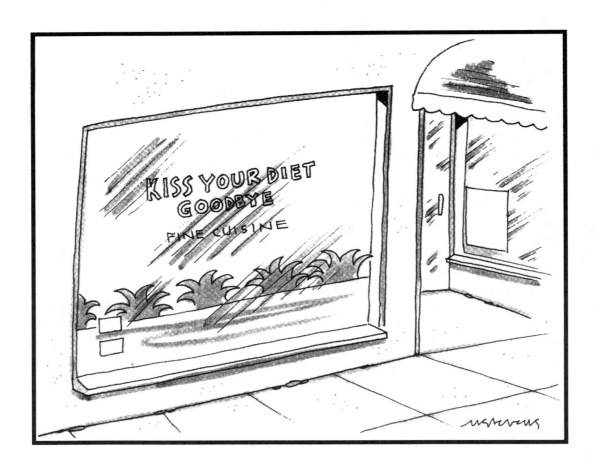

A Fault-Free Diet—Eat, Eat, Eat!

As the baby chipmunk asked his mother, "If we are what we eat, does that make me nuts?"

Tray bon. Gorging food has been a worst-cake rejection remedy since cavemen found that enemies tasted best when roasted. And the Friar's Club continues that tradition. "We only roast those that we love." Don't believe it.

*My mother's menu consisted of two choices—take it or leave it. —**Buddy Hackett***

S-cargo: Dr. Andrew Weil, in *Time* magazine, theorizes that indulging in food cravings—like ice cream and candy—is an expression of chronic stress. It's also an addiction like drugs and alcohol. It is estimated that 41 percent of all women soothe their worries with food. Then they worry about weight control. The underlying problem, he says, is a disturbance of dopamine, the neurotransmitter that mediates pleasure. He suggests not worrying about it, just switching to healthier recipes like sorbet instead of ice cream. "A better strategy," he claims, "is to indulge moderately, as a way of rewarding good behavior." The number of people who delight in cooking is growing geometrically. Baking is a joy. Because it takes time to purchase food, tinker with the recipe, then cook it with all the skill and ingredients of a New Orleans chef; it results in an edible benefit. The proof is in the eating, and you can share it for praise.

You know you're a redneck if you think fast food is hitting a possum at 70 MPH.

Don't choke on this: In our culture, we associate foods with emotional events, and many feel so addicted to foods they even attach a moral component to eating. An insatiable appetite, like Prader-Willi syndrome, is a rare genetic defect that can cause morbid obesity and related illnesses such as diabetes, choking, and internal complications.

Fish and quips: One of the best types of foods to eat when you're depressed is fish—rich in omega-3 fatty acids. Once or twice a week a seafood diet of salmon and tuna will help your self-esteem because it lowers blood pressure, slows age-related mental decline, and lowers your propensity for heart disease. That's why it's aptly known as brain food. There is also comfort food. Dr. Joyce Brothers cooks such foods she remembers from childhood—like tapioca and rice pudding—and confirms that comfort food does comfort.

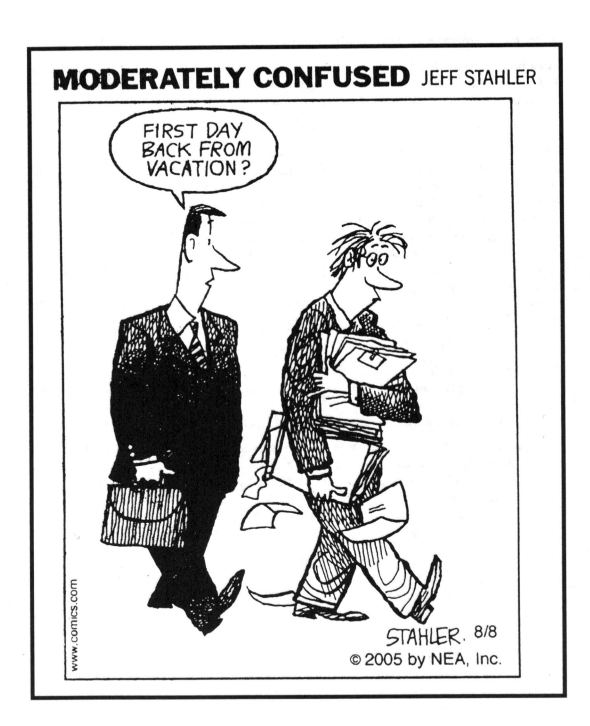

Industrial Strength Solution—
Getting Back to Business

The secret to success is to start from scratch and keep on scratching. **—Dennis Green**

Trash talk: The media is a voracious provider of trash, because large segments of the population live to eat it. Over diligent search for gossip is remorseless, relentless and borderline psychotic. So when fashion model Kate Moss was secretly photographed on a cell phone camera snorting a line of white powder, the world's press printed and reprinted that photograph, along with "what happened to Kate?" stories for weeks. Immediately, all her clients and million-dollar fashion contracts were cancelled. Then the press eagerly waited for her *mea culpa* press release spin that would create weeks of more stories. But, according to A.A. Gill of *Vanity Fair,* "Moss did nothing. She said nothing. There was no contrite press release. No TV chat with a tame interviewer. No tears. No excuses. She didn't dignify a single word." Her motto: "Never explain. Never complain."

Hide the manure: According to Gill, Moss's zip-lip lack of cant underlined her refusal to be responsible for society's woes. She was a fashion model, not a role model. With no more fodder, the press left her alone. Slowly her clients and photo gigs came back, in fact stronger than ever. "By instinct or design," wrote Gill, "Moss understood the lesson from our clamorous, cheap-talking, opinion-clogged age—that less is more." When you have the opportunity, shut up and get back to business.

In the midst of the Monica Lewinsky fracas, Hillary Clinton said that for Christmas she got a new dog for Bill. She said it was the best trade she ever made.

No self-interest: Get back to putting the customer first. Find out what's "in it" for him. Then, sell it to him. Don't let any salesperson take "no" for an answer. Tell your customer, "Let me talk to my boss, because I'm not authorized to lose this deal."

When the towing gets guff: There is a downside to getting too close to your business prospects. In business, the theory has been to become so personal with your customer that she becomes your friend. But that creates its own problem when the customer, who has confided in you, becomes so embarrassed by her indiscreet confidences that she soon breaks off the relationship completely.

I have an 18-year-old daughter. Her name is Alexis. I chose that name because if I hadn't had her, I'd be driving one. **—Robin Fairbanks**

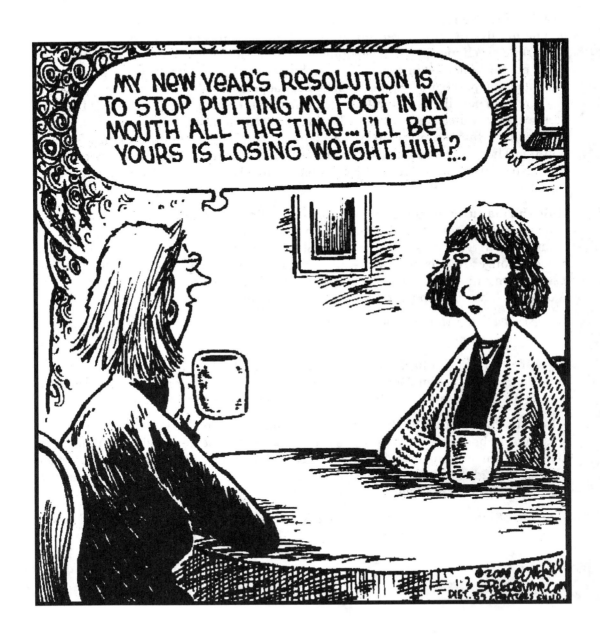

Good Guys Finish Last—
The Hungry Finish First

Our character is shaped as much by our failures as it is by our successes. **—John Gray**

Character is easier kept than recovered. It's like those who see the beauty of the rose and not its thorns. Not everyone agrees.

My mother always said that a rose is the perfect symbol of romance. It dies after a few days, its pretty petals fall off, and all you're left with is the ugly prickly thing.
—Maureen Murphy

Make realistic commitments. Go out on a limb—that's where the fruit is. Purposely put yourself under pressure. Athletes know they perform at their best when the need for success is at its highest. So do public servants. One of the best current examples of this dictum is Barack Obama, who suffered his first political defeat when his opponent noted he wasn't "black enough," because he had a black skin but a white family. Obama sunk into his own private racial displacement through alcohol, pot, and cocaine. Trying to recuperate, he kept being turned down for dates with Michelle, a girl he eventually married. "What do you do when you have a very assertive guy who keeps asking and asking?" she asked. "What you do is give in." Now confident that he had the girl he needed, Obama decided to "live up to his father's expectations" by using Lyndon Johnson's character as a role model. "I was fascinated by Johnson's hunger—desperate to win, please, succeed, and dominate," he wrote. Obama, a brilliant speaker who became a courageous politician, admits he had to be pushed into public service, "not always because I thought it was fun, but because it was necessary." Today, a Senator and a Presidential candidate, he is so overexposed he makes Paris Hilton look like a recluse.

They say such nice things about people at their funeral that it makes me sad that I'm going to miss mine by a few days. **—Garrison Keillor**

Dear John: Elton John admits he originally put on his "good guy" persona out of need, rather than benevolence. "I was a drug addict for 16 years," he admits, "but then through luck, I was given a second bite of the cherry. It was important to get involved with activities that would keep bringing me down to earth with a thump." He dresses on the humor side when he performs. "Look," he explains, "I'm stuck at a piano, which is not a glamorous instrument. It's a nine-foot wooden plank. You can't utilize it like a guitar, you can't move with it, so it's necessary to make people look at me."

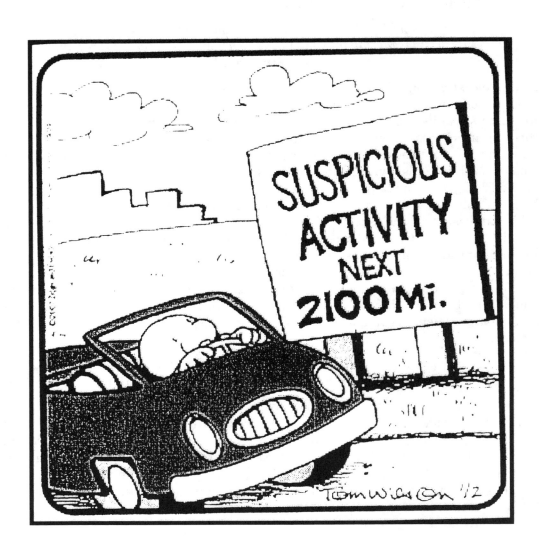

Exit Strategies—Hitting the Road

When I went to college, my parents threw a going-away party for me, according to their letter. **—Emo Philips**

Get out of Dodge: With the song "Get Out of Town Before It's Too Late, My Love" playing softly in the background, let's consider a rejection so devastating that you're considering getting out of Dodge City immediately. As an example, Maya Lin designed the Vietnam Veterans Memorial, one of the greatest anti-war statements of all time. Although it was the unanimous choice of the jurors, Lin had to endure such a long period of hateful criticism from well-placed protesters ("It was designed by a gook") that, immediately after the construction was completed, she left Washington, swearing never to return.

The reason so many people want to get away is the difference between the optimist and a pessimist. The optimist proclaims that we live in the best of all possible worlds, and the pessimist fears this is true. **—James Branch**

One step at a time: It may be therapeutic to deal with a shattered relationship by moving away from an ex-loved one. But the sad awareness is that it won't immediately undo the pain because you must still pack memories. O.J. Simpson, whose tainted past still infects everyone he touches, moved to Florida, as far from California as he could go and still be in the U.S., in order to blend in with the Cuban population. The better part of prudence is to find a place for you and the family that makes long-term sense. For example, Maui in Hawaii sounds like an escape to paradise, and it is, except for a few serious considerations: (1) it is so expensive that if you can afford living there without further income, why are you leaving town in the first place, and (2) if you're over 50 and need immediate specialized medical attention, the closest major hospital is four hours away, even if the med flight helicopter from Honolulu arrives on time.

I joined the Army because I was 18 and bored with the seventh grade. **—Robert Hawkins**

Roads scholar: Joining the Army or the Foreign Legion and eliminating your anger by fighting for your country has been the theme of many movies, many of them B—as in B or not too B. Military recruiters, however, know that difficulty in school is a strong argument for enlistment. Join the Navy and see the world, join the Air Force and fly into the wild blue yonder (just where in the hell is yonder?), and join the Marines and never be left behind. You'll never be surprised how quickly a previous disappointment in private life will disappear as you're digging a foxhole.

I love my husband. I love my children, but I want something more—like a life. **—Rosanne Barr**

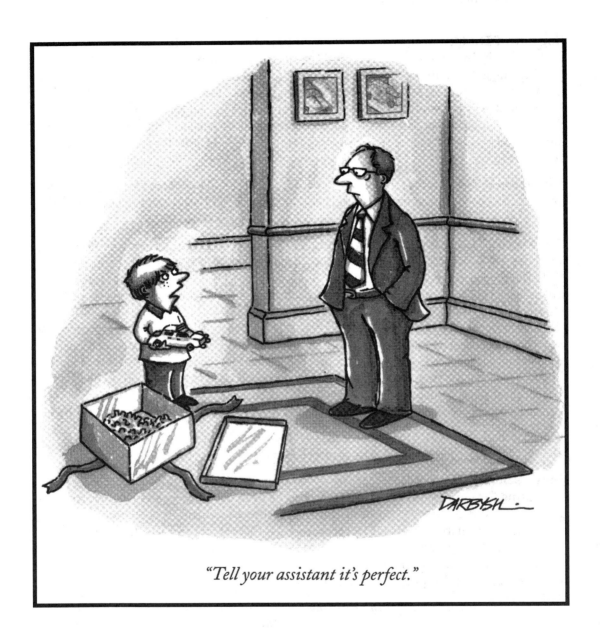

"Tell your assistant it's perfect."

A Gilt Trip—Buying a Gift for Someone

*I'm open for any gift that will get me though the night: prayers, tranquillizers or a bottle of Jack Daniels.—**Frank Sinatra***

License to thrill: Few solutions are as immediate and inexpensive as the simple strategy of buying a gift for someone else. Whether it's a book or flowers or a diamond bracelet from Tiffany's, you're suddenly an admirable benefactor and the recipient of physical hugs and written thanks. Holiday gifts are always appreciated, but if you give a gift off-seasons, it will be far more memorable—and so will you. What's equally important is the card or note you insert in the package. Clever Hallmark cards are impersonal and soon end in the trash. On the other hand, your own effort with words of affection or humor can earn you a long-term exhibit on the most treasured billboard in the house—the refrigerator door.

*I like gifts that include food, because the second day of a diet is easier than the first. By the second day, I'm off of it. —**Jackie Gleason***

Book it: When actress Brooke Shields went public about her postpartum depression after the birth of her new baby, her news drew criticism from many in the media that she was just trying to gain sympathy, not help. Knowing how hurt she felt when the public turned against her, she now takes the time to help friends through their difficult periods by buying books or connecting them with websites that contain quality material about their particularly problem. "None of this indicates that I am crazy or abnormal," she said. "You can't count yourself a friend unless you're willing to do something positive when others are in need."

*I learned about sex the hard way—through books. —**Emo Philips***

You've been Warren'ed: When Warren Beatty wants to finesse rejection during a media interview, he impresses the journalist—male or female—with a special gift. He buys lunch—not a fabulous Lutece extravaganza, but a pizza. He knows it's more seductive when you meet at "this little Italian joint I love." He's careful, cagey, watchful and deliberate. His additional gifts, during an interview, are intended to be personal—a previously untold secret, an eye-to-eye intimate look, a boyish enthusiasm about your life's tribulations, and ending not with a handshake but a warm embrace. Does it work? Following an interview, writer Amy Wilentz gushed, "He represents not only the enduring qualities of male sexuality—beauty, wildness, and a hunter's sense of unswerving pursuit—but also the more ineffable qualities that establish celebrity—stimulating intimacy while maintaining enormous distance." Obviously, Amy's pizza came with a lot of crust.

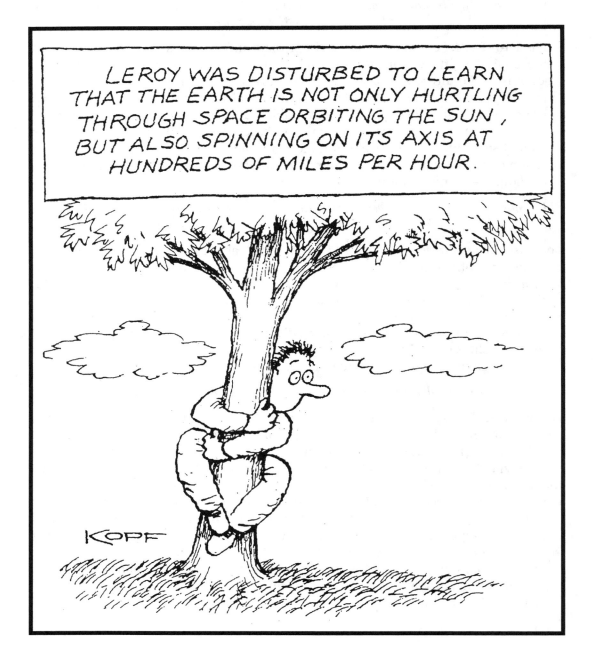

The Meek Shall Inherit the World—
Going with the Flow

When you have an elephant by the hind legs and he is trying to run away, it is best to let him run. **—Abraham Lincoln**

Go with the flow: Never believe either your own press clipping or any personal hubris that you can change the world. You can dispute the facts like the polar bear cub, standing on an iceberg, who said to his mother, "I don't care what they say, I'm cold." Or stop worrying about the cub and just buy yourself a good fur coat.

The meek shall inherit the earth, but they won't avoid probate. **—Don Haupman**

He who wears his heart on his sleeve will have one helluva cleaning bill: As you rush along the road of life, some days you're the bug and some days you're the windshield. So temporarily pull off the road and clean up your act. Both are good ideas.

The meek shall inherit the earth, because they're too stupid to refuse it. **—Jackie Vernon**

Remarriage is the triumph of hope over experience: Worry is seeing your failures in exaggerated forms. There is no such thing as a perfect plan, and so you cannot expect perfect results. Expect obstacles. Be flexible and go with the flow or roll with the punches, whichever simile is easier to imagine.

We were poor. If I wasn't a boy, I would have had nothing to play with. **—Redd Foxx**

Every crowd has a silver lining: One of the best pieces of advice I ever received was when I became a professor and the dean warned me not to fight the system, because I would never win, but to use the system. After all, we sing "Take me out to the ballgame" and we're already there!

"I come from out west, where men are men and women are women. And you can't ask for a better setup than that." **—Red Skelton**

"Oh, yes, you can. I come from New York where men are men and women are men, too."
—Robin Williams

Familiarity breeds: Or if you want to constantly change things, just imagine all the trouble you'll run into. Like if mother's milk were a health hazard, where would you put the warning label? And what would you do if you actually saw McNuggets on a chicken?

I'm not sure of the definition of déjà vu, but I have the feeling I've seen it before.

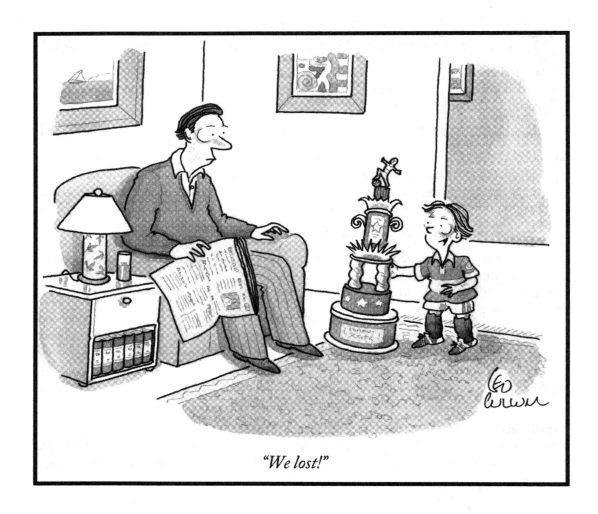

"We lost!"

The Small Stuff—Lasting Pleasures

Have confidence that if you've done a little thing well, you can do a bigger thing well, too.
—Joseph Storey

Wash out: Cavemen didn't ponder the state of happiness. They were more concerned with avoiding sudden death. Today, however, happiness is cognate with luck. When Hurricane Katrina washed away Kevin's belongings in New Orleans, he lamented that the only thing he had left was his experiences. "I value those more. They can never blow that away from me." In a recent national survey 57 percent said experiences made them happier than material things. Daniel Gilbert, author of *Stumbling on Happiness,* wrote: "One barrier to pursuing experiences in our society is that people feel they should have something tangible to show. But, in truth, the fond memories of your experience should be valued more."

The erectile dysfunction drug Cialis warns that if your erection lasts longer than four hours, you should tell your doctor. Tell my doctor? At my age, I want to tell everybody.
—Mel Helitzer

Absorption: You are at your happiest when you are absorbed in what you are doing. If you're working on a large number of projects, the rejection of any one of them becomes less important. Instead celebrate your frequent successes and victories, even when they're small. Daniel Kahneman, a Nobel laureate, reported that people's top four favorite parts of the day were sex, socializing, dinner and relaxing. Our bottom four, he claimed, are commuting, work, childcare, and housework. So much for domestic tranquility.

Bernie, an 85-year-old friend in Miami, called, "I've got cataracts in both eyes, my hearing is gone, my memory is so bad I can't remember where I put things, and my hands shake all the time. But I've got great news today. My Florida driver's license was just renewed.

Call no man happy until he's dead: When she was 22, actress Ann-Margaret was a reckless sex kitten, with leading roles (they never called her "a leading lady") opposite Elvis Presley and Hollywood's most famous pelvis thrusters. Then she descended into alcohol abuse, took an overdose of painkillers that nearly killed her as well as the pain, had a nearly fatal 22-foot fall from a stage in Lake Tahoe, and endured more than one motorcycle crackup. In America, wrote Nancy Griffin, show business gypsies are not supposed to be resilient. But Ann-Margaret credits her Swedish family with a positive attitude combined with love, discipline and robust genes. She wrote: "Where I came from, if someone said they were going to do something, they did it."

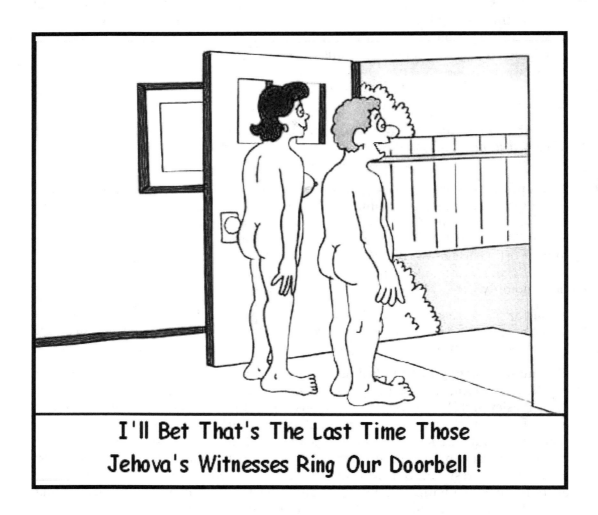

Trivialize Rejection—Life Goes On

Mel's hell: As a profession, public relations is most effective as a person-to-person communication. So in my advanced PR classes at Ohio University, I help students overcome their fear of public speaking by insisting that they not answer questions from their desk but go to the podium at the front of the classroom and give their report in two minutes—without notes. The first time, they're often caught off-guard and are petrified by the fear of failure in front of 50 of their colleagues. By the end of the quarter, having performed a dozen times, they seem impervious to fear. Some, in fact, acquire an insatiable hunger for the attention and applause. "You can't do everything perfectly the first time, nor should you try," claims Linda Sapadin, author of *Master Your Fears*."If you do, you'll not only feel overwhelmed, you'll never venture into unexplored territory to find out just what your abilities are."

Give each rejection a low value number: Rate your rejection importance on a scale of one to ten. In the beginning, you'll consider giving most rejections high numbers. But as you start to evaluate each one and rank it with other events in your life, the numbers will get lower and your spirits will increase by degrees.

I've got a doctor who has more degrees on his wall than he has on his thermometer.

Home cooking: If you worry that you can't be happy all the time, you're not being very realistic. Instead of saying "I don't want to be where I am," flip the attitude to "I'm happy with what I've got, but I know I can do better." Don't make any public rejection remarks or write a letter that will embarrass you years later. Read the letter over, discuss it with a friend to evaluate its worth, and then trash it. "Measure twice, cut once" is a well-known garment-maker slogan. It fits this body of work, too.

My father is in semi-retirement. He goes halfway to work, and then he thinks better of it and comes home. —**Tommy Koenig**

All in the family: "Why are senior citizens often categorized as either little old ladies or grumpy old men?" asks Ellen Graham of *The Wall Street Journal*. You have two choices to avoid the label: you can make peace with forgetfulness or impulsive road rage, or you can laugh them off and be a sit-down comedian. For example, retirement no longer sounds the death knell of romance. In senior-citizen centers, as in Florida, the number of newlyweds over 65 has increased six times in the last few years. Women over 70 still seek "Mr. Right," defined as "any man with money in two banks who is ambulatory."

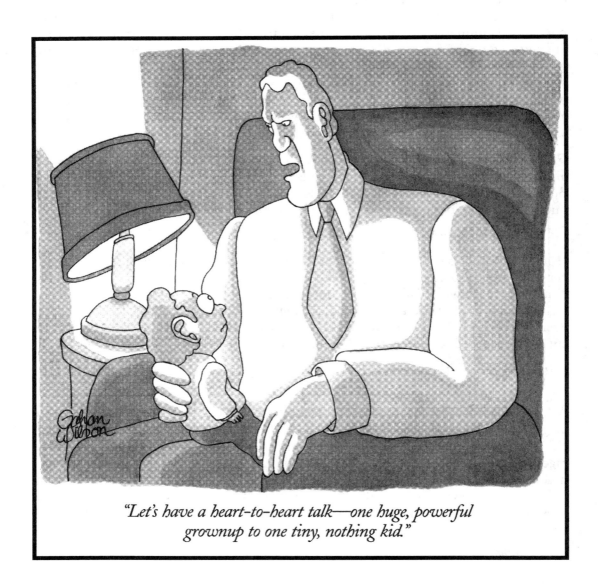

"Let's have a heart-to-heart talk—one huge, powerful grownup to one tiny, nothing kid."

Seeing the Whites of Their Lies—
Face-to-Face Conversations

Education is the ability to listen to almost anything without losing your temper or self-confidence. —**Robert Frost**

Lip service: Today's college students' fluency in interpersonal communications has reached a new low. Their conversation repertoire seems confined to such expressions as "It's kinda like . . . " "I don't know," "It's cool," "You know what I mean," and "Awesome." They have adopted the street language of inner-city kids by calling males "man" or "dude" and females "ho's," babes" or "bitches."

The good word: "Civilized conversation is like a Frisbee," wrote Margaret Shepherd, co-author of *The Art of Civilized Conversation,* "You can catch it, spin it, and toss it to the next person." You don't need charm school, but you must appreciate that it takes practice to speak with sincerity and style. Here are three absolute requirements to be persuasive in face-to-face meetings: (1) accept that other people are most interested in talking about themselves, (2) that their intent is not to appear foolish, and (3) that they wish to be recognized as being very important. For example, when confronted with bad service or food in restaurants, complain on the spot. According to Alex Susskind of Cornell's School of Hotel Administration, a face-to-face discussion gets action more quickly.

MC introducing beautiful girl at reunion dinner, "And now let's hear from the classmate who's changed the most since graduation. You may remember her better as George Ferguson."

Eye bawling: Ever since Radio Shack management got a public black eye for informing 400 employees that they were being terminated through an impersonal email ("Unfortunately, your position is one that has been eliminated in order to improve our long-term competitive position in the marketplace."), corporate executives have learned that layoff notices need to be done in person. This has been a double blessing for employees. Having a face-to-face meeting helps you plead your case against furloughs and for promotions. There's a lot of preparation needed for success when asking for a raise. *Fortune* magazine reports that less than 1 percent of the people who ask for a raise get it right away, but don't let that statistic deter you from the big picture. A private meeting, during which you demonstrate diplomacy, loyalty, and responsibility, will raise your profile with your supervisor. Don't expect her to automatically know about your ability.

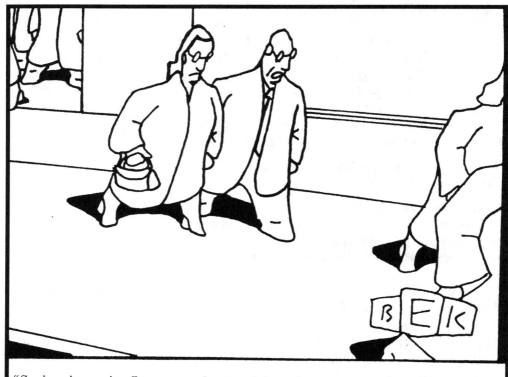

"Seeing it again, I was newly struck by whatever you thought about it."

Casablanca for the 90th Time—
Weeping at Old Movies

I asked my husband, "Why don't you make passionate love to me like Brad Pitts does?"
And he said, "Are you kidding? Do you know how much he gets paid to do that?"

Tearjerkers: The term works. Old sappy Hollywood films' main purpose—after making money—was to wring out your emotions through sadness, rejection, love, patriotism, and comedy. Rejection was the most common emotion of all.

Terribly pleased: When you feel rejected, 90 minutes of sympathizing with Ingrid Bergman while she's on again and off again with Humphrey Bogart is a lot more effective than a 50-minute stint on a psychiatrist's couch. Unfortunately, today the main element in million-dollar blockbusters is fear and, utilizing computerized effects, traumatizing your mind. They're not only bigger than life, they're dirtier than life. In the old days, performers used to play parts. Now they just reveal them.

*When my wife and I watch romantic movies on TV, she insists upon turning out the lights. Then when the movie inspires me to make love, my problem is to overcome her ability to hide. —**Jonathan Katz***

Silent Scream: There are scores of old movies that soothe, not abuse, no matter how many times you see them. That's the reason why films like *It's a Wonderful Life* and *The Wizard of Oz* capture major audiences in reruns year after year. They specialize in happy endings. Life can be beautiful. Old comedy films, like comic page cartoons, not only can make your present problem seem ordinary but may actually help you fight serious illness. Norman Cousins, in his book *Anatomy of an Illness,* claimed that hours laughing at films with the Marx Brothers, the Three Stooges, and Bugs Bunny cartoons ameliorated the pain he felt from an incurable brain cancer.

I'll never understand why people go to the movie theater to talk to each other. The idea is that you paid to see and hear someone do something better than you can do yourself.
*—**Rita Rudner***

Remote control: DVD films can be borrowed from libraries. You can dress any way you wish, you can be alone or in a group, and you dictate the time of the performance. One-third of people surveyed said their living rooms, now with large-screen HDTV, are their ultimate movie location, and popcorn at home is a lot cheaper and healthier.

*I always loved stage business, so when I retired, I developed an act at home of exaggerated mimicking and clowning. I was such a hit with our friends that my wife started charging a four-dollar cover and a two-drink minimum. —**Shecky Green***

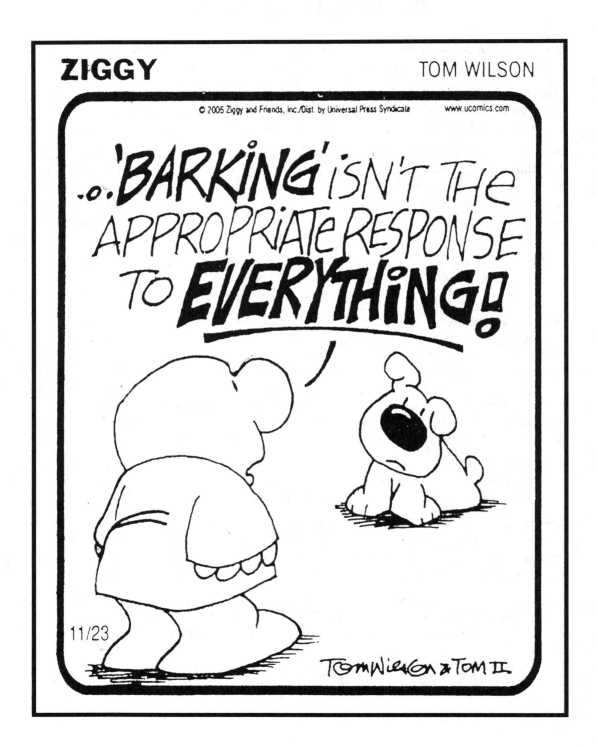

No Go!
26 Commonly Considered Actions—Not Recommended

There are many strategies for coping with rejection that are so onerous that no analyst would recommend them. But, on the other hand, no examination of rejection would be complete without their listing and examination. Depending on the circumstances, they have also proven successful to those who like to live dangerously.

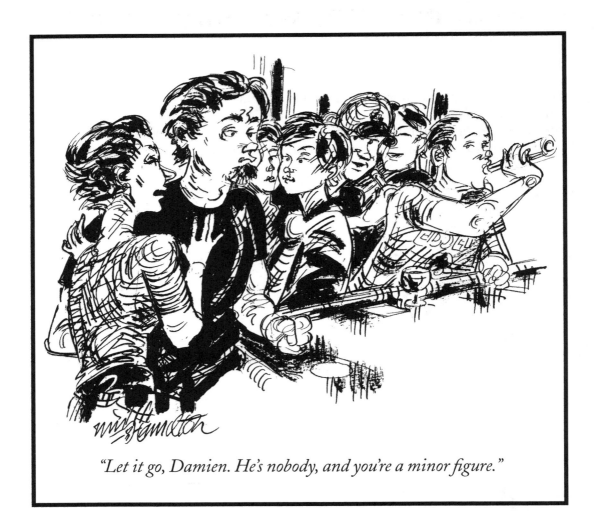

"Let it go, Damien. He's nobody, and you're a minor figure."

Demean the Critic—Obviously the Worst Idea

He only acts mean. But down deep in his heart, he's thoroughly rotten.

Screw Me? Screw You! Because it's the first response that you will feel, we recommend that it be the first response you ignore. The impulse to strike back, to demean the qualifications of your detractor, is instinctive. To sue, to go public with your own accusations may be therapeutic, and may also be exhausting and—to the delight of your lawyer—very expensive.

He had this four-inch wound in his head that was always open. It was called his mouth.
—Mel Helitzer

My fart belongs to Daddy: The most demeaning and consistent critic in playwright Clifford Odets' life was his father, L.J., who brutally chastised his son's every play and action. When Odets separated from his wife, L.J. wrote him a public letter, "I'm ashamed of you. You are the dumbest chunk of humanity I have ever come in contact with. You are all ass-backwards and sitting on your brains." Odets internalized these public excoriations by depicting characters in his plays based upon his father, as a gangster, a womanizer, a puissant Hollywood mogul, an idiot, and a loafer.

A little heat is a big price to pay. If you have a public persona—published author, pro athlete, politician, businessman or entertainer—a new, uncensored brush fire of criticism can come 24/7 from Internet blogging and there's nothing you can do to stop it. The Internet has allowed anyone with a computer to pretend to be an expert on anything. "No matter how uninformed, unintelligent or unrestrained people may be, they can declare themselves authorities and everyone else complete idiots," claims Clark Gerhart in *Time* magazine. And the major problem with attacking your detractors is that criticism they level at you gets wider circulation when your rebuttal is also public.

I had a civil ceremony. His mother wasn't invited. **—Phyllis Diller**

Professional critics: Generally media critics, teachers, coaches, and panel judges are professional in their disciplines. Your mother-in-law is not. Even so, the way you respond to criticism says a lot more about you than the sour remarks tossed at you. Learn from criticism despite your initial disagreement. Cooperating responses, such as "I'm sorry you're disappointed. Let's see what I can change to make it acceptable" are magical.

Open sass-a-me: Accusing a critic of impaired communication skills only adds fuel for their fire. Following a negative story in the *Columbus Dispatch,* the provost at Ohio University wrote a scolding letter to the editor demanding more favorable stories about her college. Within two months after her disparaging letter, the paper ran more than 25 stories about the university on their front page—all of which were negative. Coincidence? Maybe.

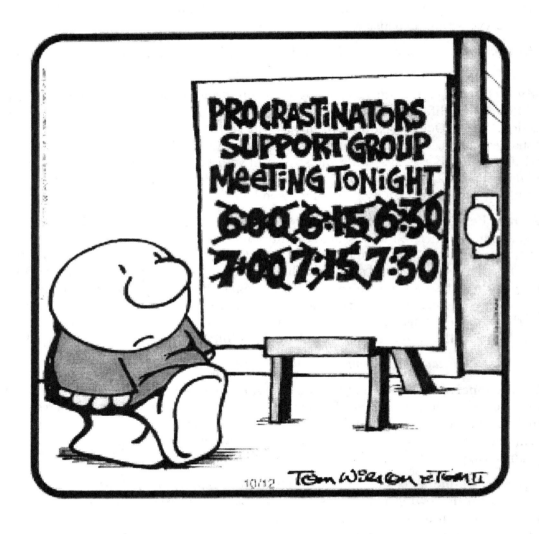

Resting on Your Laurels—Procrastinating

*My mother said, "You'll never amount to anything if you keep procrastinating." I said, "Mom, just you wait." —**Judy Tenata***

My favorite four-letter word is "next": "I'll do it tomorrow" is the proverbial promise about action delayed. Fearing the pain involved, we avoid problems by procrastinating, hoping the anguish will just evaporate. According to M. Scott Peck, author of *The Road Less Traveled,* "Some will go to extraordinary lengths to avoid facing problems by trying to find an easy way out, sometimes building elaborate fantasies to the exclusion of reality. Unfortunately, the tendency to avoid the emotional suffering inherent in problems is the primary basis of mental illness." Helen Keller claimed, "Character can not be developed in ease and quiet. Only through experiences of trial and suffering can the soul be strengthened, vision cleared, ambition inspired, and success achieved."

*Procrastinate now. Don't put it off. —**Ellen DeGeneres***

Win or lose: Every time you do something, you can learn from it and find a way to do it better next time. "What you do right now," said Anthony Robbins, "is what will shape your destiny. The only thing that's necessary to make a positive change is to begin to learn that it is possible to change." And the fastest way for you to change is to demand action as if you were a boss tearing into a subordinate. Without action, you keep regurgitating the rejection scenario like sitting through a bad film that was terrible the first time you saw it and that you can't bear to see again.

*The first time I saw Deep Throat, I thought it was disgusting and insipid, and I thought it was disgusting and insipid the third and fourth time I saw it. —**Mark Shatz***

Get out of bed: The only time success is assured, say pessimists, is if you plan to do nothing. But optimists point out that if you stay in bed, you'll certainly die there. You can avoid procrastination attitudes by breaking your assignments into small parts and giving yourself an award for each accomplishment. If you can't reward yourself with a vacation, try a dinner, a manicure or some new clothes. Avoiding a lifetime decision such as getting married, or having children, or saving for a major future expense can create major espousal concerns. But the faster a decision is made the less anguish it can cause. One of Edgar Guest's most quoted poems is "Tomorrow." The last few lines end with:

The greatest of workers this man would have been
Tomorrow
And the world would have known him had he ever seen
Tomorrow
But the fact is he died and faded from view
And all that was left when he was through
Was a mountain of things he intended to do
Tomorrow.

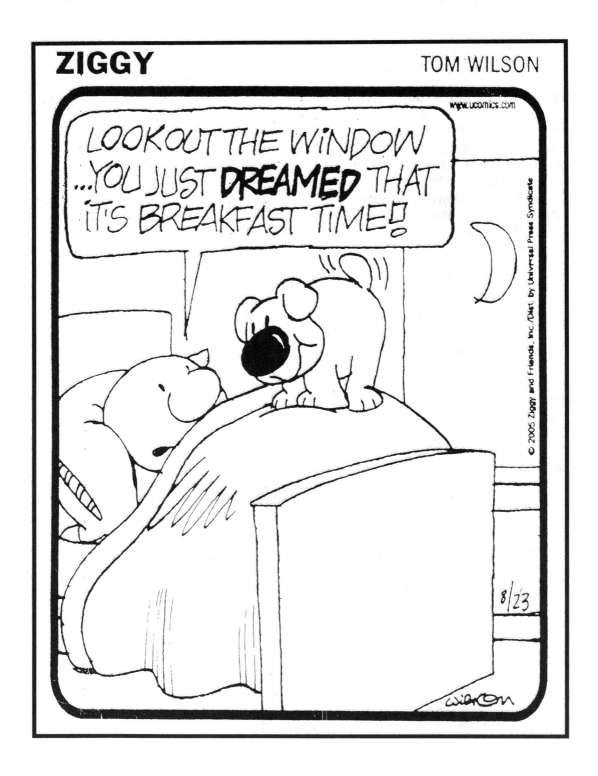

Stop the World, I Want to Get Off—
Staying in Bed

*They say the early bird catches the worm. Frankly, I'd rather stay in bed, then take a shower and have a toasted English muffin. —**Shirley Lipner***

Mary Mapes was fired by CBS for helping produce a devastating *60 Minutes* segment with Dan Rather that ridiculed President Bush's National Guard record based upon documents that could be not be authenticated. Within days, she was jobless, friendless, and felt worthless. She succumbed to an ever-present, aching fatigue. She slept for hours. "It was one way," she wrote, "that I was able to escape the catastrophe that I had wrought in my career. Nothing seemed to have any real impact on me anymore. I kept watching the clock. Is it time for another pill yet?"

The escape syndrome: When there's a major rejection, there is a common first remedy that is to shut the door and stay in bed all day. Psychologists call this the escape syndrome and, in truth, there is nothing drastically wrong with it, including the crying jags. When you don't want to talk to anyone, when you don't want to go out in public and when you don't even want to look yourself in the mirror, bed is one of the most consoling places to be. In your own horizontal sanctuary, no one asks questions and there's no retribution. Few people will know about it, and all the rest don't care.

Enough already: While staying in bed is certainly an immediate and tempting retreat, it can also be one of the worst. It flirts with depression. The trouble starts when this escape hatch is used more than a week. By that time, the next logical step is to seek some kind of qualified help from a physician, an analyst, a religious counselor, a respected friend, or a physical trainer to work out your anger by pounding every muscle in your body. You'll know you've reached the stage of acceptance when you wake up one morning and say, "Enough already. Let's get on with life. I'm better than all this."

Weapons of mass distraction: There's also nothing wrong with being fat. Tyra Banks was a top model who decided to retire at 40 and ease off the required disciplined diet, punishing exercise and avoidance of the gourmet backstage grub available at her TV show. Within months she gained 40 pounds and the tabloids generated international buzz by labeling her "Tyra pork chop." She was not ugly or disgusting, just plump, but her photos were being airbrushed, her contract with Victoria's Secret was canceled, and the criticism affected her sleep and her personality. So she decided to endorse the benefits of a full-sized figure, lauding the artwork of Rubens and the talent of Judi Dench. Her combativeness took the fashion world by surprise, and she joined Fergie, the Duchess of Kent, and Kirstie Alley as spokespersons for healthy women who don't need to hide big breasts, wire hips, and bouncing stomachs. Who could argue with that?

The last time I visited my doctor, he showed me an article in the Journal of the American Medical Association which claimed that teenagers who masturbated frequently in bed had fewer prostate problems when they became senior citizens. I said, "I'm 80 years old and now you tell me?"

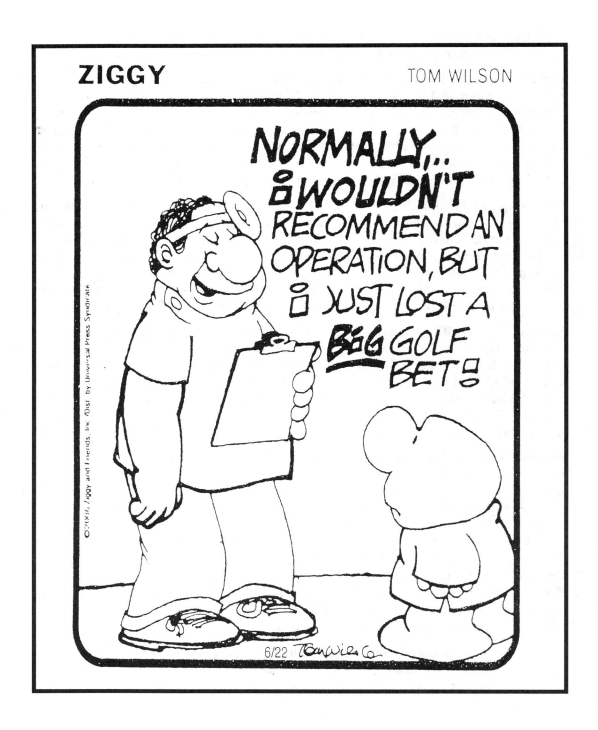

A Friend in Need—
Not Necessarily a Friend in Deed

George invited one of his best friends to his vacation home on an Adirondack mountain lake. While they were swimming, a poisonous Copperhead bit his friend on his penis. George immediately cell-phoned the local hospital, 50 miles away, and asked the emergency room doctor what he should do. "Put the wound in your mouth," said the doctor, "and suck out and spit out the poison for at least five minutes. Then get him to the hospital as fast as you can." George, perplexed, asked, "Isn't there any other way?" "No," shouted the doctor, "and you'd better start immediately or your friend is going to die." George snapped off his cell phone as his friend, withering in pain, gasped, "What did the doctor say?" George looked at his friend for a moment and said, "He says you're going to die."

Is this guy necessary? The need for friendship has changed dramatically over recent generations. Years ago, it was considered necessary to have a vast array of friends. A few years later, many claimed that four or five friends were quite fulfilling. Today, research indicates highly cultivated people get along with just two friends.

My father makes money the American way. He trips over stuff and sues people.
—Dominic Dierkes

A friend in need, when you are constantly bitching, whining, or crying, could be your worst rejection consultation. Friends may be convenient, but they are rarely experts, they are not objective and they are not especially brilliant, or why would they want to be friends with a rejection prone person like you in the first place. Friendships can also be demanding. If you get, you've got to give. "So some friends," claims Joseph Epstein in his book *Friendship: An Expose,* "need solace without being remotely in trouble. Like strict schoolteachers, they require perfect attendance. Constant demands, by either party, can be tedious, tiring and only fitfully rewarding."

For every rejection these days there's a support group of friends, most of whom have one solution, "Meet me at the bar."

Forget about a friend in deed, talk to a professional analyst. Save your friendship from fatigue. It is best to be quiet on topics that impose a lot of personal detail. Too many medical details can cause repugnance at the lunch table, too many emotional problems take too long at the water cooler, and too much complaining will turn off co-workers who were originally sympathetic.

If you lend someone $20 and never see that person again, it was probably worth it.

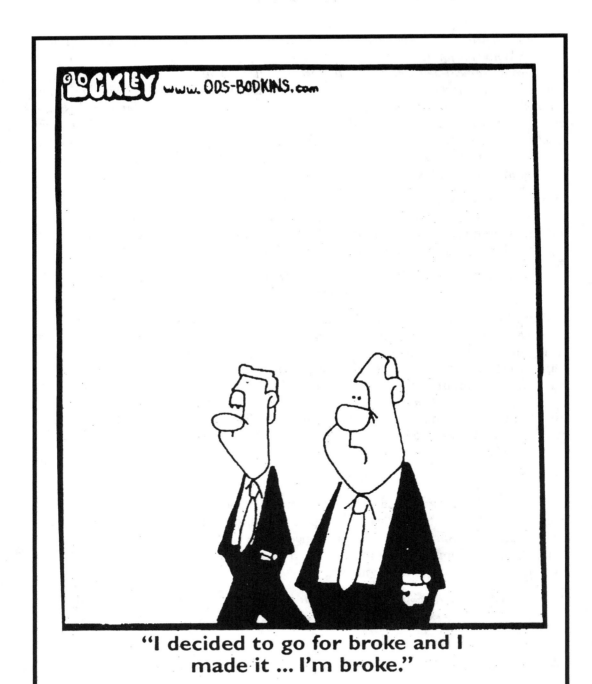

Double or Nothing—Maximizing Your Losses

The best way to double your money is to fold it over once and put it in your pocket.
—Kim Hubbard

Double your bets: After rejection is no time to complain that haste makes waste. Set a high rejection threshold. It's akin to high-stakes gambling, when you're behind at the tables, you're tempted to double your bets just to get even. Smart people don't gamble because they're already even.

Americans spend $300 billion every year on games of chance, and that doesn't include weddings. **—Argus Hamilton**

Like an athlete, remember that a temporary loss is not the end of the season. Be patient. No tantrums. Stay in the pool and tread water; you can't drown that way. Things will be clearer after a short dunk.

The trouble with life in the fast lane is that you get to the other end in an awful hurry.
—John Jensen

And, there is always next year. No supporters in any sport are more loyal than baseball fans of the Chicago Cubs, who haven't won a World Series since early in the 1900s. "Hey," said announcer Harry Carey, "anybody can have a bad century." Las Vegas stickmen know the odds on each roll of the dice or turn of the roulette wheel are exactly the same as the last one—and it's all in their favor. So when losing bettors start to panic by doubling up their bets, the house gleefully rubs its itchy palms. And then there's the long-suffering cardiac patient who refused a transplant saying he'd already had a change of heart.

A wife wins the lottery, rushes home and says to her husband, "I'm rich, so start packing." "Wonderful," shouts the husband, "What should I pack, for warm weather or cold?" "Make up your own mind," answers the wife. "Just get the hell out of here before sunset." **—Red Buttons**

Miss communication: John Ashbery, arguably the most important living American poet, had his first poems rejected by *Poetry* magazine with a single-word reply: "Sorry." But ironically, despite the fact he didn't believe he was truly qualified, he made his first paychecks from teaching and writing poetry criticism. "I feel I could be making a mistake that would cause somebody unhappiness," he said. "Who am I to say whether it's any good or not?" Other critics are not so ambivalent. A former Ashbery student, John Yau, received one of his poems back with a footprint from an editor who dropped it on the floor and stepped on it.

A beautiful call girl walked into my hotel room, and said, "Oh, I'm sorry. I must be in the wrong room." I said, "You're in the right room; you're just twenty years too late."
—George Burns

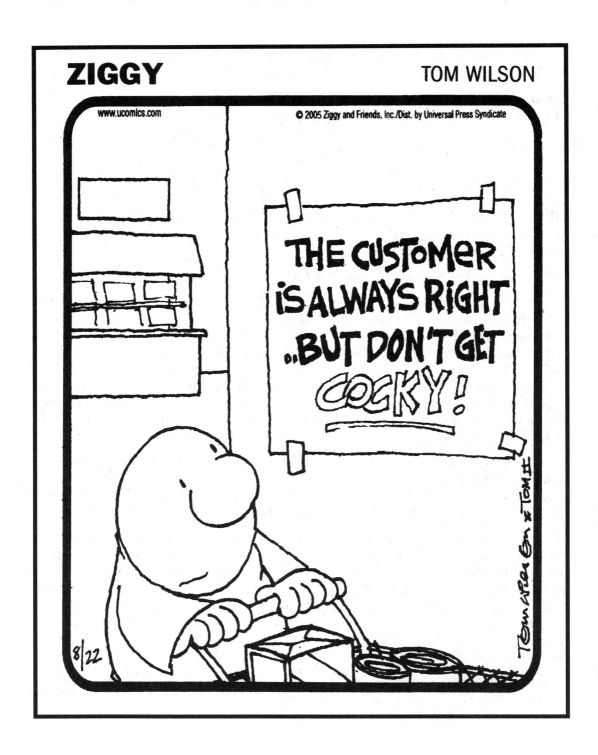

Power to the People—Disassociation

If at first you don't succeed, then skydiving isn't for you.

Isolation: They say that once you understand the Morse code, a tap dancer will drive you crazy. Well, anger is a primal instinct, but withdrawing from a battlefield may not be the shrewdest maneuver. Leaving the room or going silent by being unresponsive and avoiding immediate verbal retort may drive your reviewer crazy with fear.

When a woman says to you, "The last thing I want to do is hurt you," what that obviously means is that it's on the list, but that she has some other things she wants to do first. **—Mark Schiff**

The older you get, the less depression you feel when rejection hits. You learn to accept what happens and look at the upside of most situations. "Positive thinking," claims Gene Pitney, "is a wonderful fan and it can blow away the rain on any given day." An example is the story of Staci Columbo, a VP of marketing for a Las Vegas casino, who was pregnant and planning to get married when her fiancé, suffering from depression, committed suicide in front of her. She rushed into counseling for the rest of her pregnancy to defeat her anger. After the birth of her child, she gave up dating because she didn't want to confuse her son by rotating a lot of men in and out of her life. Instead she turned to pets and founded a kennel to house abused animals. "It's my way of dealing with negativity," she said. "Animals teach us about love, and I'm able to get smarter about life as I go along. I've stopped trying to be perfect."

I'm currently dating a girl with no self-esteem, because if she had any, she'd leave me.
—Devin Dugan

Kurt Vonnegut said that a person must suffer rejection in order to write a novel. On the other hand, being hurt by the failure of a current friendship should never forestall the attempt of another intimate relationship. Looking for new friends is better than opting out of society. It is not braggadocio to believe you are valuable to other people. The feeling that you are essential and important reinforces your self-esteem and you can make it happen.

For twenty years, Cristobal Balenciaga was the premier couturier in Europe's chic fashion industry. Royal princesses insisted on wearing his gowns and dresses, and a delicious effusion of "ravishing and inspired" creations set the tone for glorious critical reviews. Then one year, when his showing was lambasted by the effete fashion media, Balenciaga's infallible ego balloon was deflated. It was like a genie that could not be put back in a bottle and discarded on the beach. He spent months planning his revenge. The next year, he refused to show his new collection during the precise dates dictated by the Chambre Syndicale de la Couture but insisted on a private showing in Paris a month later, forcing his peers, buyers, and journalists to expensively trudge back to Paris. He not only got his petty revenge, but his independence earned him exclusive coverage in every style column and magazine, wrote Judith Thurman.

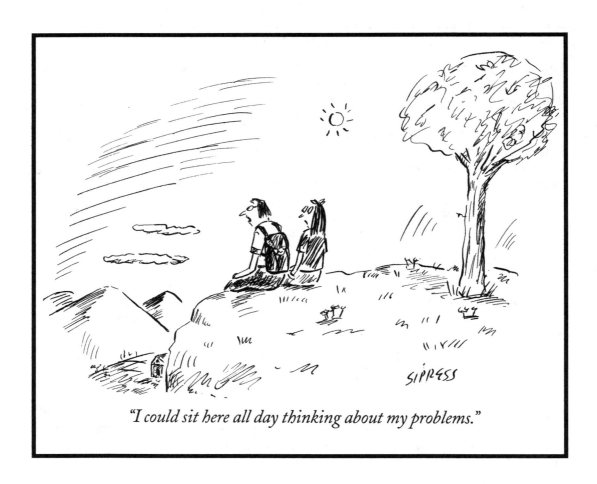

"I could sit here all day thinking about my problems."

Include Me Out—Physical Laziness

Even if you're on the right track, you'll get run over if you just sit there. **—Will Rogers**

It's called prioritizing. By doing something each day, you can judge your own worth. You waste time with simple distractions: making lists, gabbing on the phone with friends, or shopping. In this movie, home is your main stage. Your act is to care for it endlessly: the grass always needs mowing. It may look greener on the other side, but it's just as hard to cut. You lighten your load by delegating—after all, isn't that the reason you had kids. Or you are convinced that if you wait long enough, nature will care for itself. But then the bathroom has leaks, your closets need straightening and your refrigerator and oven need cleaning, so you get off the couch to keep the walls from falling. You are convinced that your sacrifices will eventually lead, if not to sainthood, at least a step above welfare. The worst baggage of this *faux* laziness scenario is that you might insist your family join the ensemble and, even worse, that you have avoided the opportunity to feel truly proud.

I went to a bookstore and asked the clerk where the Self-Help section was. She said if she told me it would defeat the purpose. **—Dennis Miller**

Take out the garbage: "When I have the blues," claims Wynonna Judd, "I start organizing my house. I start with the basics, the sock and underwear drawers, and move up the stuff chain. The cleansing process works on my mind, too. The more clutter I remove from the physical world, the more my emotional load lightens." Every day we collect and save more stuff. It gets buried along with our other junk, but it's always there. It is necessary to renew yourself physically and emotionally by cleaning out the clutter you no longer use because of wear, size or style. Donate it to the Salvation Army, or to another favorite charity. Don't make a big ceremony about it, because each item may have a memory that you may feel like retaining. Dump it. The only way to create a new beginning is by being ruthless. "Without clear space to grow in," wrote Bernie S. Siegel, "you can not come out into the light of the day."

One hen said to another chicken, "I enjoy laying eggs, and my farmer gets 75 cents a dozen." And the second hen said, "When I lay an egg, I push and push with all my might to get the biggest egg possible, and my farmer can get 80 cents a dozen for my eggs." "Look," said the first hen, "for five cents a dozen it doesn't pay to strain yourself."

Salt shaker: Kristen Bell's best friend died in a car accident when she was 18. She took to her room and refused to come out until her parents suggested she start acting. "Losing someone should make you grateful for what you have," they told her. So the Hollywood star started work with Invisible Children, a charity that helps kids who have been kidnapped. She claims, "Compared to them, I've learned to take criticism with a grain of salt."

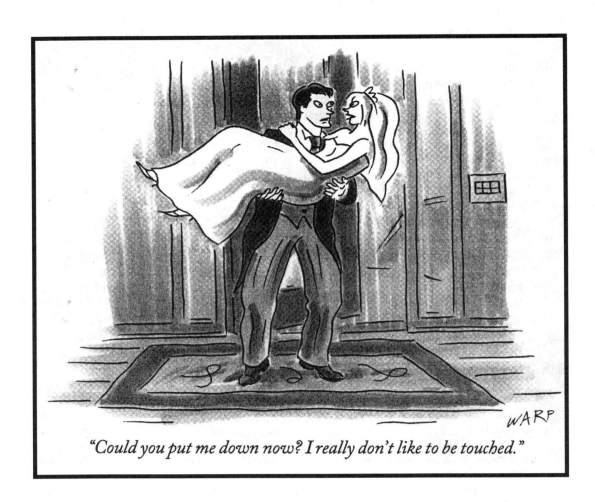

"Could you put me down now? I really don't like to be touched."

The Comeback Fib—Negative Thinking

I'm a pretty good judge of people, which is why I hate most of them. —**Roseanne Barr**

If you must first live in peace with yourself, then forget about "loving your neighbor as yourself." Most cultures accept a tactile relationship—touching and embracing—as a common expression of love or friendship. But what if you suffer from germophobia, as comedian-TV host Howie Mandel does? Because he has an aversion to germs (he even shaves his head of all traces of hair), he can't bear to even shake hands, let alone embrace anyone. In an industry where air kisses are common, Mandel finds it excruciating to participate in any touching affection. "I know I'm not going to die or get sick," he reported, "but when my hand is touched, you have no idea what I have to go through."

Going out with a jerky guy is kind of like having a piece of food caught in your teeth. All your friends notice it before you do. —**Livia Squires**

Supervisors, regardless of title, unconsciously judge your integrity on seemingly innocuous behavior. One candidate for a major executive position showed up at a dinner interview with his mistress. He was immediate disqualified because the CEO felt that if he was cheating on his life partner, he wouldn't hesitate to cheat his company.

We are what we pretend to be. So we must be careful what we pretend to be.
—**Kurt Vonnegut**

The admonition to do unto others as you would have them do unto you is in every religious tradition. Ethics is about getting outside of our own selves. Ethical behavior, claims Dr. Bruce Weinstein, is not just the right thing to do, it enriches our lives as well. Positive identity and positive intimacy are like tango dancing partners. You cannot have perfection without both being in sync. Taking the low road, as an arrogant Martha Stewart discovered, is the worst possible choice.

An optimist sees a challenge in every calamity. A pessimist sees a calamity in every challenge.

Stress occurs often when you need to adapt to change. Even advertising slogans with smiley-faced logos for lottery tickets properly claim, "You can't win if you don't play." Rewritten, the line could read, "You can't win if you don't think positive." Distress is bad stress. "Eustress" is the word for good stress, a condition so rare that even the word is rarely used. Wasted stress is your demand to know all the negatives from friends who are not willing or qualified to tell you the unvarnished truth. Better to be the proverbial optimist who looks for, but rarely finds, that pony in the muck pile.

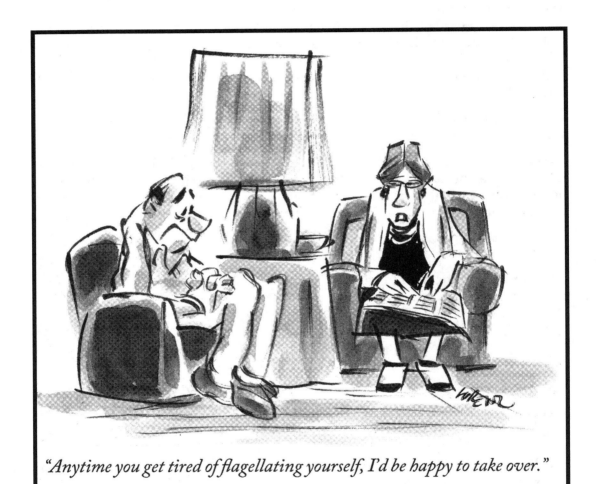

"Anytime you get tired of flagellating yourself, I'd be happy to take over."

Let's Have a Party—Pity Me

The hard luck kid: When you try to avoid pain, it creates greater pain. So throwing yourself into your work or spending more time with your children has been a favorite device for navigating through post-split hurricane depressions. First NBA star Lamar Odom's six and a half-month-old son died of sudden infant death syndrome. That tragedy was followed by the death of his mother, then he was robbed at gunpoint, and finally a rash of injuries sidelined him from play for weeks. Overcome with grief, Odom wanted to quit the pros, so his teammates painted the face of his late son on a giant-sized t-shirt and hung it in Odom's locker. "At first I was angry," he told them, "I didn't want pity." But under their encouragement, he was able to turn doubt into a process of accomplishment. "I kept saying, I'm a good person, and good things will happen to me. I believe there's a karmic action in life that works for you."

Numb the pain: Another outlet is a pity party. Jennifer Aniston's marriage to Brad Pitt broke up soon after front page photos appeared of her husband and his new girlfriend, Angelina Jolie, frolicking on a beach. As her anger, hurt and embarrassment all blended together, her immediate catharsis was to walk to the ocean's edge and scream. After that was her realization that "What doesn't kill you makes you stronger." Her longer-term resolution was to throw little pity parties for herself. Surrounded by a small tribe of friends, she was able to maintain a very positive outlook. The only party subject was humor and the only party evidence was a few bottles of wine. The evenings ended in a good mood, and the beverages helped bring sleep more quickly.

"I like parties," claims Troy Body. "I think friends exist for our pleasure. They are like neighbors in a small town; they already know your business. I tell them everything. I have dessert parties, Saturday afternoon parties, parties before a party and happy-to-be-alive parties." Open your best bottle of wine, eat until you're dizzy and be grateful your nosey-ass friends care enough about you to share your sad times. Then, suggest that each guest share a story (true or not) about "one my worst decisions," or "how to be happy, though married," or "one of my wildest sexual experiences." By the end of the evening, with many outlandish anecdotes having been told, you'll realize the insignificance of your own dilemma. And they'll think you cared enough to listen.

Pity me: Another pity party is writing a heart-rending book that camouflages your grief as evasiveness posing as courage. That's what author Joan Didion did when, within a short period, her husband died from a massive coronary and her teen-age daughter died from pancreatitis. Her eerie memoir of self-pity was her road back to sanity. "Having lived through the worse," she wrote, "very little can happen to me now. We tell ourselves stories in order to live."

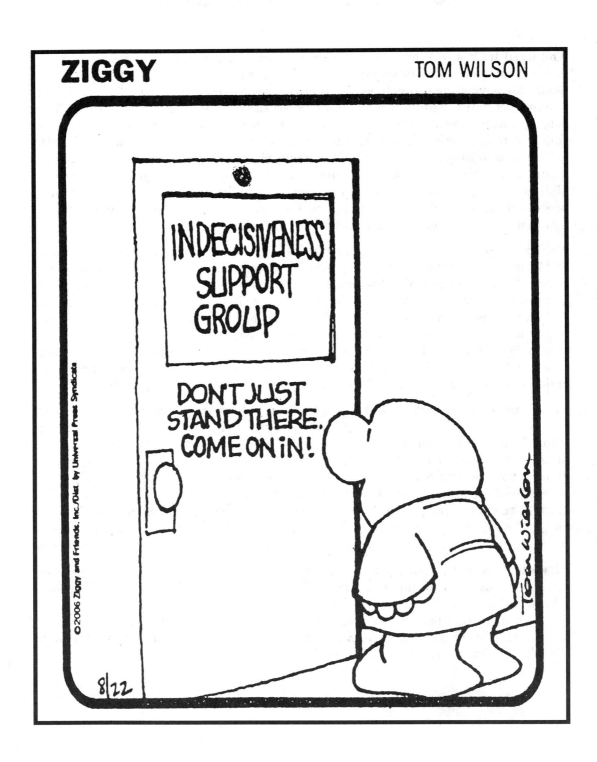

Better Than Doing Nothing—Meditation

The only reason some people are lost in thought is because it's so unfamiliar territory.
—Paul Fix

A thought for today: In meditation, you get in touch with your immediate concerns. The Japanese have an expression *wabi sabi,* a specific aesthetic awareness that translates to "less is more in an attentive melancholy state." The Japanese culture, difficult for Westerners to understand, appreciates simple food, simple design, and pastoral scenic pleasures. This attitude is particularly valuable if one assumes that things can always go wrong and therefore life should be approached with wry skepticism.

Whoever thought up the word "mammogram?" While I'm meditating, does it mean I'm supposed to put my breast in an envelope and send it to someone? —Jan King

You don't have to be a monk. Meditation is one of the oldest forms of rejection therapy. Thinking is what it requires and thinking is what makes it develop so many benefits:

(1) It involves deep breathing and the most popular physical manifestation is yoga.
(2) It helps you connect to a comforting place.
(3) It demands quiet reflection on your thoughts, not reality.
(4) It is particularly helpful for elderly people who want to keep their minds fit and alert.
(5) It helps you have a clear, nonemotional view of thoughts passing through your mind.
(6) It helps you delay reacting to destructive thoughts and then helps you let them go.
(7) It takes a lot more from your mind and puts a lot less on your plate.

A Freudian slip is when you say one thing, but mean your mother.

Yoga bare: Petra Nemcova won fame modeling a string bikini on the cover of *Sports Illustrated*'s swimsuit issue. But she believes it was spiritual human yoga that saved her life. "Every person goes through difficult moments and each time there's a choice," she claimed. "Either it makes you weaker or stronger, putting even more meaning into your life." While on a vacation, she was swept away by the infamous tsunami that killed 300,000 in Southeast Asia in 2004. She recalls flailing for her life in the wet, eerie darkness in less than 12 feet of black water. Yoga taught her to remain cool, and suddenly, without even trying, she surfaced and escaped a drowning that took the life of her boyfriend. "Instead of fighting the world," she said, "it's best to just trust and let things happen."

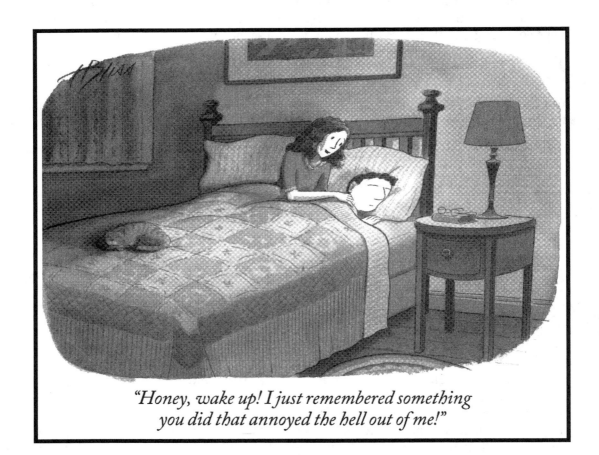

"Honey, wake up! I just remembered something
you did that annoyed the hell out of me!"

Ranting and Raving—Never Stop Complaining

Complaining burns calories. That's why skinny women are always such bitches.
—Debbie Kasper

Another day, another holler: One of the fastest ways to turn your friends off is to be a constant complainer. You think they're really interested in your problem and that they don't have problems of their own. You're wrong. 50 percent of them don't care and the other fifty percent are glad you're getting what you deserve.

I personally think we developed language because of our inner need to complain.
—Lily Tomlin

What a bitch: Some companies will penalize you for grumbling on the job. They are convinced that moaning is bad for company morale. But Lucy Kellaway of the *Financial Times* claims moaning helps her get through the workday. "It lets me blow off steam and express exasperation at the same time." She even offers four guidelines for bitching etiquette.

(1) Set a quota, no more than 24 minutes a day,
(2) Lighten your complaints with humor,
(3) Whine only to those on your level. Moaning upward irritates the boss and complaining downward finds people who aren't interested,
(4) Practice using the expression "Ah, the hell with it." Then, get back to work.

The only thing worse than going to your friends and family is going public in print. It used to be that publicizing "your side of the story" by writing a story for the local news, or having a press conference if you're especially famous, or even writing a letter to the editor would get public sympathy, maybe even a bright idea. Remember that by making waves, the most visible gets criticized first. By defending your position publicly, through letters or even through threatening legal action, you're spreading the bad news faster. Only lawyers are guaranteed to make money at a lawsuit. And not everybody respects them.

A man complains to his Pastor, "Pastor, something terrible is happening. My wife is poisoning me. What should I do?" The Pastor said, "Let me talk to her."
A week later, the Pastor calls, "Well, I phoned your wife. For three hours she complained the whole time. I've never heard anyone complain so much. Now, do you want my advice?" The man said, "Oh, yes!" The Pastor said, "Take the poison."

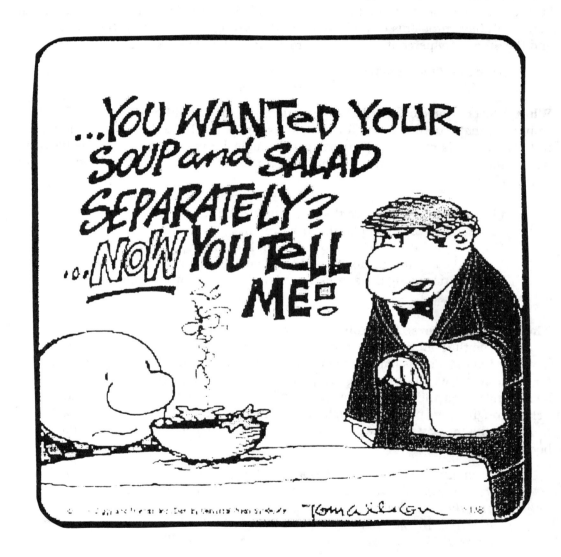

Barking Up the Wrong Me—Blaming Others

It's not only whether you win or lose, but where you place the blame. —**Harry Bressler**

Find a scapegoat: It is not ethical to avoid blame by deflecting it elsewhere. It just begs more trouble, and rarely provides long-lasting gratification. We've learned from high profile cases, like Watergate, Martha Stewart, and the Iraq War, that a cover-up can have a worse result than the crime. By pointing the finger at others, you encourage the media or opponent organizations to investigate and find there's little truth in your charges. Then, you're not only a culprit but also a liar.

My dad asked me, "Have I been a good father?" I said, "Dad, you've been the best. Why do you ask?" And he said, "I wanted to make sure the way you turned out is your fault."
—Stu Trivax

Out of context: The most common attempt to shift blame is the claim "I was misquoted," or its twin brother, "My remarks were taken out of context." Both are such a common practice among celebrities and in Washington that communication specialists just assume it's the most conventional thing to do. History is replete with misappropriated, misquoted, and misattributed catchphrases. Humphrey Bogart never said "Play it again, Sam." Sherlock Holmes never trotted out his signature "Elementary, my dear Watson," and Cary Grant never uttered "Judy, Judy, Judy." Even though it's been pointed out over and over in biographies that it was Benjamin Franklin, not Mark Twain, who predicted, "There are only two certainties in life: death and taxes," and it was Red Sanders, not football coach Vince Lombardi, who first bellowed, "Winning isn't everything, it's the only thing," these botched quotes will remain in the public perception forever. The second most common shift of blame when a program goes sour is the practice of pointing to an innocent underling as the victim ("He was authorized to sign my name, but not in this case"). Certain professions, such as accountants, engineers and husbands, are paid to accept the blame.

A fool and his money were lucky to get together in the first place.

The kiss of death: Why do we always blame another when we've made a lush bankroll and then pitifully lost it? Unless we were a lottery winner, we found it was easier to lose it than it was to win it—but it will always be someone else's fault. *Everybody Wants Your Money,* wrote David W. Latko, and rascals will try to steal it with high-risk business investments, unparalleled embezzlement or just efforts to marry you. Mike Tyson earned and lost more than $400 million in his boxing career, and Michael Jackson's multi-million-dollar habit of personal spending ran amok. To keep from being exploited, you need to stay away from liquor, Shylocks, and beautiful blondes.

As the farmer said to his infertile cow, "I'm sorry I gave you a bum steer."

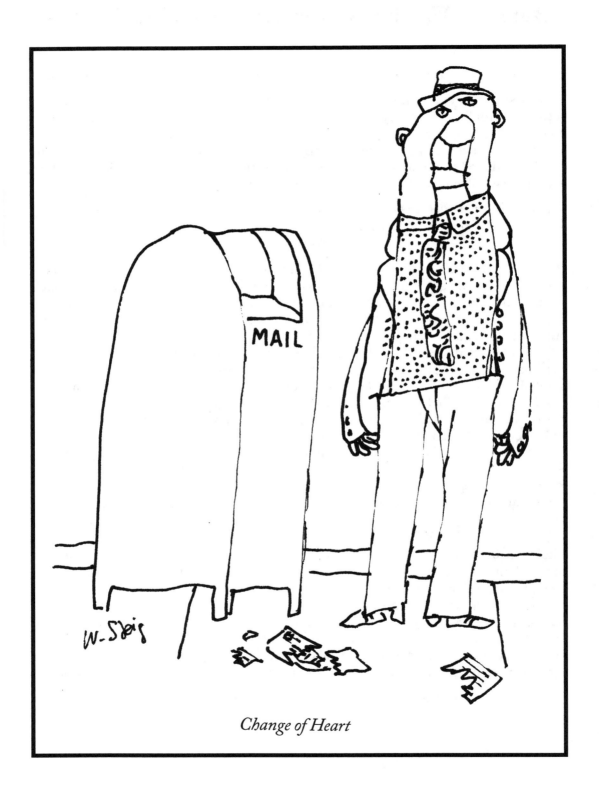

Change of Heart

Take Out the Trash—
Apologizing, But Not in Writing

The easiest time to eat crow is while it's still warm. The colder it gets, the harder it is to swallow. —**Farmer's Almanac**

Oops! Apologies will ameliorate 80 percent of all crises, but it very important in how they're done. Harry Whittington, a friend of Dick Cheney, took the heat off the Vice President by publicly apologizing for getting his face in front of Cheney's shotgun. The media world laughed at such a ridiculous gesture, but the apology worked and the story was over.

I talk to my mother every day, because hearing how delusional I may become makes me appreciate every day what I have left of my sanity. —**Tami Vernekoff**

Did I say that? The best advice is that when you are in deep doo-doo, howl your apology as quickly as possible before you're the target of a howling lynch mob. Mel Gibson, the Dixie Chicks, and Michael Richards discovered that while being a celebrity inflates perks, it also inflates damages when vocalizing against the unholy trinity: race, religion, and patriotism. Portraying the part of Kramer, a klutzy, twisted-tongued lout in the TV show *Seinfeld,* Richards was discovered to be a klutzy, twisted-tongue lout on-stage as a result of a racist tirade during a stand-up routine. Richards hired one of the nation's most powerful publicists to get him on as many TV interview shows as possible to apologize. The first thing the publicist did was to send out a written statement, "Michael wants to heal the tremendous wound that he's inflicted on the American public and on the African-American community." It generally takes two years of water under the bridge to wash away that pollution.

I like to reminisce with people I don't know. —**Steven Wright**

The proof is in the writing: Expressing your regrets privately is laudatory. Even doing it publicly, if called for, can satisfy public antagonisms. But be careful when you feel it necessary to write a letter of apology. In serious cases, like when you are involved in an accidental death, it is unadvisable. Your lawyer will get hopping mad.

Trial by error: Jeanne Phillips, current author of the "Dear Abby" column at the Universal Press Syndicate, was chastised by her readers when she recommended a letter of apology to the family of a young lady whose death was caused by a drunken driver. A regret letter will not make the deceased survivors feel better but will only inflame their emotions. In fact, they may use it as an admission of guilt against the writer in court if there is a charge of homicide. Everything written in that letter can and will be detrimental to the final plea. If you feel the need to apologize, do it after the trial.

If the facts don't fit the theory, change the facts. —**Albert Einstein**

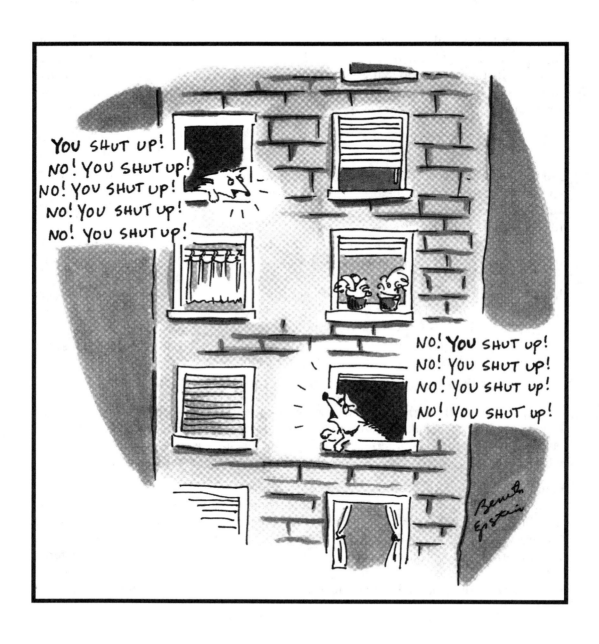

Go Public—Yelling From the Rooftops

Nobody knows the trouble I've seen, but I keep trying to tell them.

For some reason, when you're rejected you want the world to know just how angry you are. You call your spouse, kick your dog, and scream at your mirror.

"Why do I generate instant hate?" the President asked his wife. "Because it saves time,"
she answered.

Go public: The loudest way to let the world know about your problems is to believe in scream therapy. In 1970, Dr. Arthur Janov's book *The Primal Scream* changed the mechanical exercise of yelling into an art form. The act of primal scream therapy is to stand up, free the diaphragm so it has more power to scream, and scream at the top of your lungs. Just back away from anything made of glass. The therapy is dangerous in untrained hands, because it opens patients to recognizing their pain by losing control of their own feelings. The possibilities for abuse are limitless.

Lots of things have been opened by mistake, but none so often as your mouth.
—Gladys Case

Now and Zen: If you don't like screaming, then there are four effective ways to tell your side of a bitter story: (1) write a book or a major article, as ex-Hewlett-Packard CEO Carly Fiorina did in her best-selling book *Tough Choices,* (2) be a whistleblower and contact appropriate regulatory authorities, as former House pages did in the Congressman Foley scandal, (3) write to the company's customers or donors, or (4) go on the Internet. The newest media is blogging, where people bare their souls with an online diary complete with text, photos and even music. The popularity of blogs is increasing geometrically. It is estimated that 20 percent of teenagers have their own blog, and half as many adults either post their own blogs or read others. There are many downsides to Internet blogging that can have lifetime ramifications down the road. "It's a negative power, but it's still a power," claims Amanda Lenhart, a researcher at the Pew Internet and American Life Project. "Today's online bashing and its frank display of someone's personal life style can get you fired from your current job and be a scandalous record that could be embarrassing years later when applying for a corporate or government position."

After I had been married 25 years, I looked at my wife and said, "Honey, 25 years ago
we had a cheap apartment, a cheap car, we had a cheap sofa bed, and I got to sleep every
night with a hot 25-year old blonde. Now we have a nice car, a nice house, a king size bed,
but I'm sleeping with a 50-year old woman. I'm telling the world that you're not holding
up your side of things. Well, my wife is a very reasonable woman. She told me to go out
and find a hot 25-year old blonde, and she would make sure that I would once again be
living in a cheap apartment, driving a cheap car, and sleeping on a sofa bed.

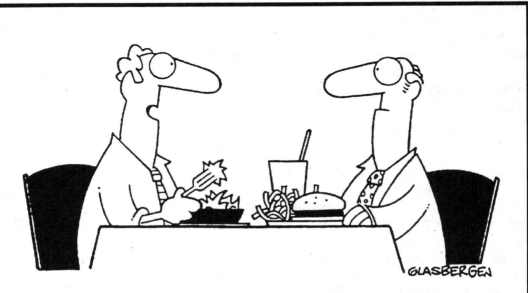

"I learned about stress management from my kids.
Every night after work, I drink as much chocolate milk
as my stomach will hold, eat handfuls of sugary cereal
straight from the box, then run around the house
in my underwear squealing like a monkey."

A Class Act—Taking Anger Management #101

As a teacher it's important to be politically correct when you're handing out grades, like telling a failing student how lucky he is that he's going to have another semester in which to get to know me better. —Mel Helitzer

Is there another word for synonym? Take a class in anger management, which teaches how to exercise more control over how to respond to stress, tension, and rejection. One of the first lessons explains how most angry outbursts by others generally have nothing to do with you. It's the steam pipe theory. The anger has been building up from previous events and you happened to be the one sitting on the toilet when the pipe exploded. It takes a strong friendship to withstand the catharsis of an angry exchange.

Adapt without compromise: How much punishment can you take? Football coach Vince Lombardi summed up his talent as someone who could tear his players down but then take the trouble to build them back up again. "You can push professionals much harder than other coaches normally do. There are some players who are so gifted that, in the past, they weren't pushed as hard as they could be." Lombardi would threaten them but also reward them. Professionals let him push them until there was nothing left. "They trusted me not to betray their interests."

We don't know the author of this great story, but we do believe it's one for the book.

When you occasionally have a really bad day, and you just need to take it out on someone, don't take it out on someone you know, take it out on someone you don't know.

I was sitting at my desk when I remembered a phone call I'd forgotten to make. I found the number and dialed it. A man answered, saying "Hello."

Politely I said, "This is Chris. Could I please speak with Robin Carter?"

Suddenly the phone was slammed down on me. I couldn't believe that anyone could be so rude. I tracked down Robin's correct number and found the problem. I had transposed the last two digits of her phone number.

I decided to call the wrong number again. When the same guy answered the phone, I yelled, "You're an idiot!" and hung up.

I wrote his number down with the word idiot next to it, and put it in my desk drawer. Every couple weeks, when I was paying bills or had a really bad day, I'd call him up and yell, "You're an idiot!" It always cheered me up.

When Caller ID came to our area, I thought my therapeutic idiot calling would have to stop. So I called his number and said, "Hi, this is John Smith from the telephone company. I'm calling to see if you're familiar with our Caller ID Program?" He yelled "No!" and slammed down the phone. I quickly called him back and said, "That's because you're an idiot!"

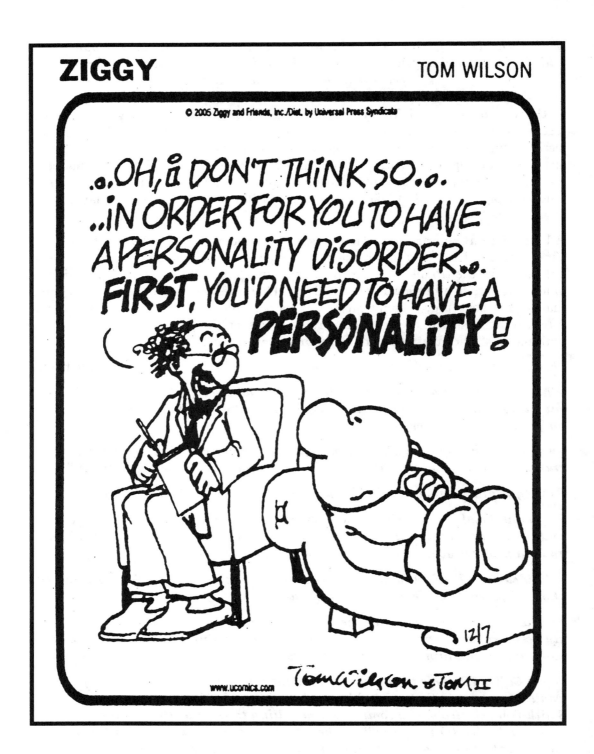

One day I was at the store, getting ready to pull into a parking spot. Some guy in a black BMW cut me off and pulled into the spot I had patiently waited for. I hit the horn and yelled that I'd been waiting for that spot. The jerk ignored me. I noticed a "For Sale" sign in his car window, so I wrote down his number.

A couple of days later, right after calling the first idiot (I had his number on speed dial), I thought that I'd better call the BMW an idiot too. I said, "Is this the man with the black BMW for sale?"
"Yes it is."

"Can you tell me where I can see it?"

"Yes, I live at 1802 West 34th Street. It's a yellow house, and the car is parked right out in front."

"What's your name?" I asked.

"My name is Don Hansen," he said.

"When's a good time to catch you, Don?"

"I'm home every evening after five."

"Listen, Don, can I tell you something?"

"Yes?"

"Don, you're an idiot." Then I hung up, and added his number to my speed dial, too. Now, when I had a problem, I had two idiots to call. Then I came up with an idea. I called idiot number 1. "Hello. You're an idiot" (but I didn't hang up).

"Are you still there?" he asked.

"Yeah," I said.

"Stop calling me," he screamed.

"Make me," I said.

"Who are you?" he asked.

"My name is Don Hansen."

"Yeah? Where do you live?"

"Idiot, I live at 1802 West 34th Street, a yellow house, with my black Beamer parked out front."

He said, "I'm coming over right now, Don. And you had better start saying your prayers."

I said, "Yeah, like I'm really scared, idiot."

Then I called idiot number 2.

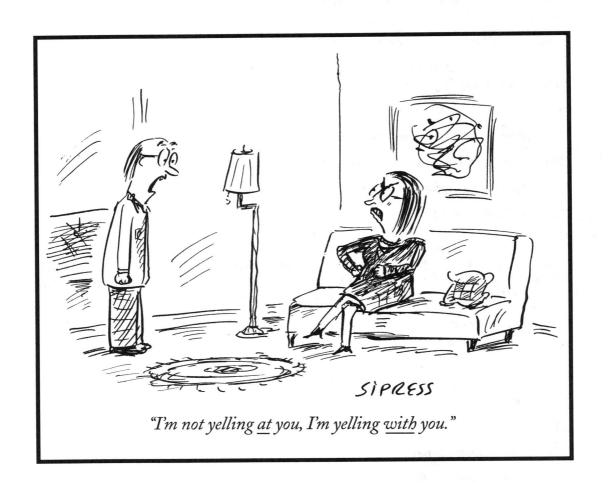

"I'm not yelling _at_ you, I'm yelling _with_ you."

"Hello?" he said.

"Hello, idiot," I said.

He yelled, "If I ever find out who you are. . . . . . ."

"You'll what?" I said.

I'll kick your ***," he exclaimed.

I answered, "Well, idiot, here's your chance . . . I'm coming over right now."

Then I hung up and immediately called the police, saying that I lived at 1802 West 34th Street, and that I was on my way over there to kill my gay lover.

Then I called Channel 13 News about the gang war going down on West 34th Street. I quickly got into my car and headed over to 34th street. There I saw two idiots beating the crap out of each other in front of six squad cars, a police helicopter, and a news crew.

Now I feel much better!! Anger management really works!!!!

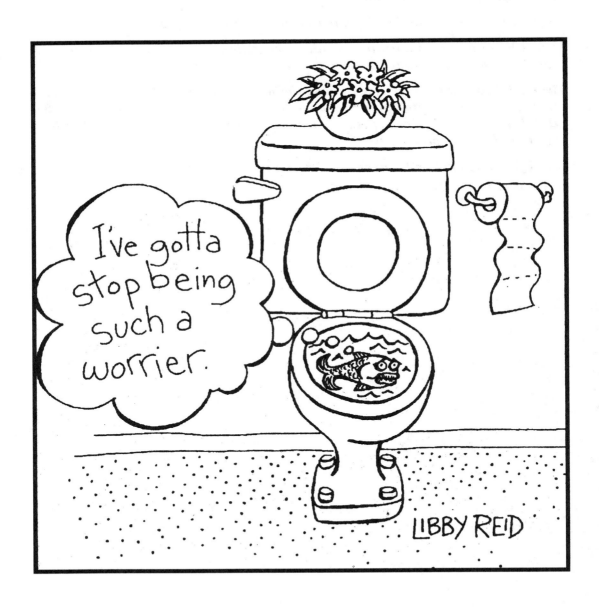

Awe Some More—Being Habitually Anxious

All human beings should try to learn before they die what they are running from and why. —*James Thurber*

Anxiety: For 4,000 years hysteria was thought to be the second most common disease after fever. Then, in 1980, the term was changed to "conversion disorder," because doctors were unable to explain symptoms that affect nearly 44 percent of all women and a slightly lower proportion of males. You are not faking this illness. If nothing else is wrong with you, claim some doctors, then maybe you've got it. Your heart pounds, your breath quickens, your adrenaline surges, and you sweat like a boxer for no reason. Something rooted in your mind is giving rise to fits, spells of crying, strange aches and pains. It could be from something simple, like taking a test or applying for a credit card. Panic attacks have no single cause, claims the American Psychological Association, but just thinking about such symptoms as elevated heart rate, heavy breathing, and unexplained nausea can bring on an attack.

I knew psychology as a child. I had a lemonade stand and I gave the first glass of lemonade away free. On the second glass, I charged five dollars. It had the antidote in it. —*Emo Philips*

Compassion: In addition, it's not a bad thing to use your own sensitivity to show empathy for others who may have the same symptoms. For example, if dependency on what others think of you leads to insecurity—that someone will criticize you or not like you, or crowds bother you so much you can't relax in jammed social settings, or if people annoy you by whistling or tapping their feet—then taking the time to learn how to be more in control of your emotions is a workable research project.

I have six locks on my door all in a row. When I go out I only lock every other row, because I figure no matter how long someone tries to pick locks, they're always locking three of them. —*Elayne Boosler*

Simple Simon Says: Some solutions seem just too simplistic—like concentrating on your breathing, or constantly seeking help from others, or celebrating your past small victories. One to avoid is "the five-second pause" rule: that before you get upset about a given situation, you wait five seconds. I just don't want to be a passenger in any car with a driver who practices that technique.

Indecision may or may not be my problem. —*Jimmy Buffet*

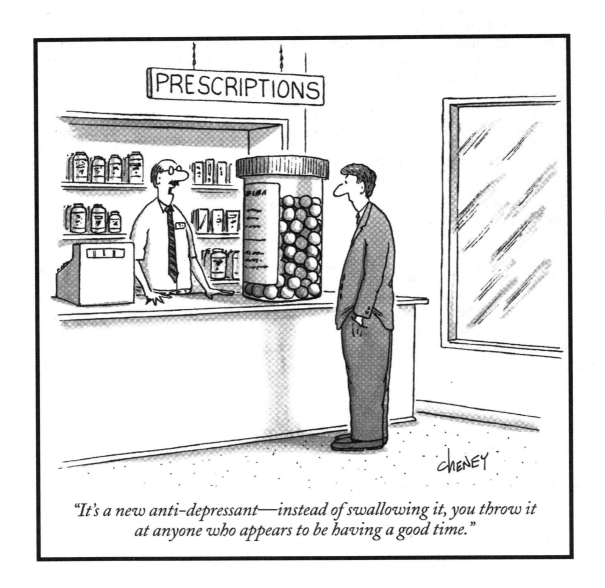

"It's a new anti-depressant—instead of swallowing it, you throw it at anyone who appears to be having a good time."

A Turn for the Worse—Looking for the Detour

If you've got a medical problem, talk to a doctor. If you've got a legal problem, talk to a lawyer, and if you've got a hot, juicy rumor talk to me. —***Lady Astor***

Spilled milk: It's easy to blame a decision made years ago for many of the major problems you have now. Feeling guilty over negative events that occurred over the early part of your life are natural. Since most of them cannot be changed, don't waste energy that can be better used to make wise decisions about events that are happening to you today. Anderson Cooper refuses to play this blame game. "Demanding accountability is no game," he claimed. "You only have so much energy and so little time. Each time you are absorbed by the disappointments of things gone by, the emotional impact weakens us as surely as termites attacking a foundation."

Desperate people do terrible things, so in high school Cooper started taking survival courses: month-long mountaineering expeditions in the Rockies, sea kayaking in Mexico, going through Southern and Central Africa by truck. "I always felt that inside me is a crystal core, a diamond nothing could get at or scratch."

If you want to see less sex in the movies, watch the film instead of the students in the audience.

The best resort: "I couldn't get pregnant," wailed writer Anne Taylor Fleming. "It was the first thing I ever failed at and the more my baby desire was thwarted, the larger the desire grew. I'm not talking about wallowing, just living beside the sadness rather than pretending it away." Fleming looked at other friends who regret their career or love choices, those who played it safe in boring jobs or lukewarm marriages for security or out of insecurity. In comparison, she discovered her lifelong regret was not the end of her world. In fact, the disappointment gave a sharp kick to life's other joys and seemed to make them all the sweeter. "It's O.K. to have a regret that's as big as the sky," she wrote. "The measure is how you live with your regrets. The best resort I know is in your mind when you to resort to forgive yourself for what you did or didn't do."

Be a quarterback: The best remedy for releasing past regrets is forward motion. Make plans for a current or future project. As in football, if the last play didn't work, think of a similar play, but include the corrections. You can't keep thinking about the last loss when the ball is about to be snapped.

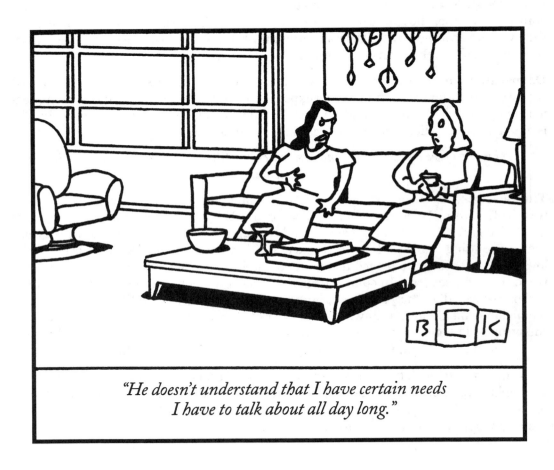

"He doesn't understand that I have certain needs
I have to talk about all day long."

The Short Fuse—Premature Ejaculation

*I went to a meeting for premature ejaculation. I left early. —**Red Buttons***

"If at first you don't succeed" may be the result of false expectations. With every crisis, resist the urge to make decisions quickly, or to speak out of turn when we are more likely to be out of breath and ideas.

*Crime of passion is a phrase that drives me crazy. A man murdering his girlfriend is not a crime of passion. Premature ejaculation, that's a crime of passion. —**Hellura Lyle***

Be audacious: By refusing to let your mind take you to a scenario of concern and dread, you can minimize the pain of being in denial, even though it may be no more beneficial than a band-aid when a tourniquet is required. You've got a doctor's appointment, but regardless of the time given you, you're likely to end up waiting in the reception room for one to two hours. To quickly dissolve the large number of patients ahead of you, wear a pair of military shirt and pants and then put on a shoulder patch that reads "U.S. Border Patrol." In the southwest, the crowd will disappear in minutes.

*I asked my wife who she fantasized about while we were having sex, and she said, "I don't know. I never have enough time." —**Owen O'Neill***

Financial retaliation is not worth its weight in gold. A famous Jewish Wall Street banker was so enraged when he was rejected as a guest at a Saratoga hotel because of its anti-Semitic policy that he bought the hotel just to fire the management. Unfortunately, his blind rage was costly, because the owners were able to negotiate a price twice the market value.

*Forgive your enemies, but never forget their names. —**John F. Kennedy***

Taboo: A societal shift toward more diversity in lifestyles has changed the rule on what is O.K. to talk about at work. It's hard sometimes to figure out what to say or what is off limits. According to Sue Shellenbarger of *The Wall Street Journal,* there are the traditional Four Horsemen taboo subjects: politics, religion, race, and gender. But that depends on what section of the country you work in. The Rednecks say, "My ball and chain stays home and takes care of our five children, the housekeeping, the cooking, the cleaning, the laundry, the ironing, and the gardening. No wife of mine is going to go to work."

When Hillary Clinton was running for President, her staff distributed a bumper sticker that read, "Run, Hillary, Run!" The Democrats put it on the rear bumper and the Republicans put it on their front bumper.

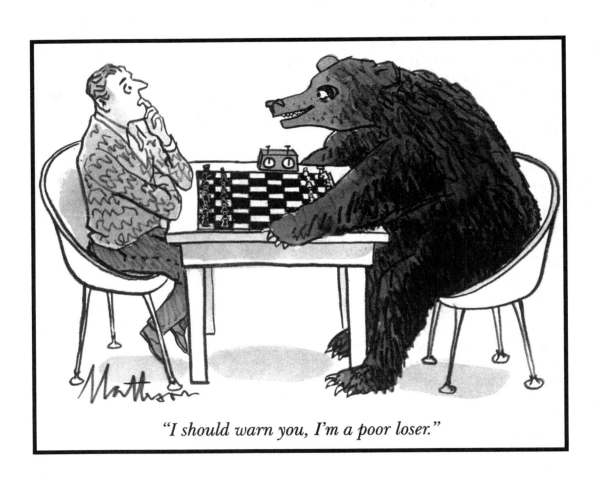

"I should warn you, I'm a poor loser."

If Looks Could Kill—Threaten Someone

*No one wants advice—only corroboration. —**John Steinbeck***

Off the beaten track: During their weigh-in and pre-fight instructions, boxers are taught to snarl at their opponent like a wild lion anticipating an attack during mating season. One of the reasons is public play-acting. A more important reason, however, is that frightening an opponent into believing you're crazy is as much effective psychology as fighters, wrestlers, football linemen, and combat Marines need to be taught. For more erudite competitors, there are the leering, menacing, mind-crushing expressions of chess masters. Winning is a mark on the score sheet. Since there are some 85 billion ways of playing just the first four moves, there is no luck involved in the game. Says grandmaster Bruce Pandolfini, "Chess is a pursuit, like music or math, where natural talent is essential. Addiction to chess is the mental equivalent of a dangerous drug, and most players behave like they are on leave from an asylum. Getting an edge with hostile glances and sinister gestures must be cultivated."

Kiss-off: "Chess is like life," said world champion Boris Spassky, but he was wrong. Chess is not like life, it's more like a state of war, which translates to death and annihilation. What top players, even champions, want to do is kill. Others wisely play defense until their opponent makes a fatal mistake. So in real life, when you're on the receiving end of threatening remarks and promissory oaths, retorts like "You'll be sorry," or "I'll get even" are exercises in futility. Silence is your best anti-toxin, and success is your best revenge. Even with that, rather than sign off with "Up yours" or "I told you so" gibes accompanied by middle-finger hand gestures, you're ahead of your adversary when you say, "I want you to know your encouragement works." And that works every time.

A sales manager said to his new employee, "I can only make one person happy a day, and today is not your day."

Never issue an ultimatum. After rejection during normal business hours, don't threaten to quit, and certainly never threaten your superiors that you will reduce your efficiency. To ameliorate the rejection, be realistic. Ask for an immediate reconsideration. Even before the next salary increases are on the table, a positive private meeting review often pays off by serious consideration not to grade you so harshly the next time. According to Joanne Cini, in her book *Kingmaker: Be the One Your Company Wants to Keep,* you should prepare a carefully written one-page summary, listing your contributions since the previous review. It must demonstrate how you've helped the company achieve its goals. Even if you are not invited to respond, a written response advances your arguments and preserves them for a grievance mechanism, for anyone who may read the review down the line or for litigation.

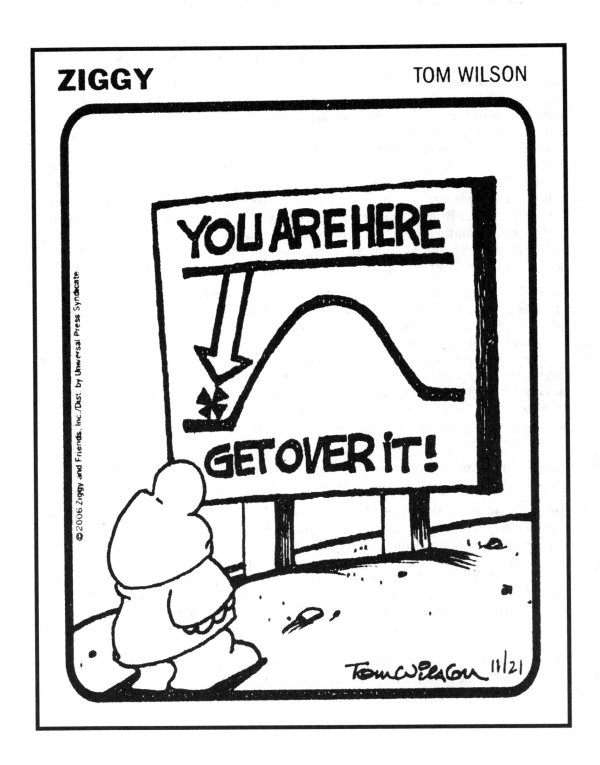

Remain Average—Staying the Way You Are

They say, "Drugs intensifies your personality." But what if you're an asshole?
—Bill Cosby

Play the averages: You can avoid goals and maintain minimum standards so you won't be compared with leaders. Consider your choices: the advantages of Thoreau's "quiet expectations" that promulgates the "status quo," or the negative Chinese adage that the nail that stands the highest gets hit first. If you let others make decisions for you, you will certainly end up being the slave and not the master.

I always thought that music was more important than sex. Then I noticed that if I didn't hear a concert for a year and a half, it didn't bother me. —Jackie Mason

Mix it up: Actress Gwyneth Paltrow compares the arc of her personal and professional life to a carnival roller coaster ride, but except for the death of her beloved father, she claims she wouldn't change anything. "Obviously, you look back and think: 'Oh, that probably wasn't the best script, or boyfriend or whatever,' all the time. On days when it's really challenging or goading, it's really depressing. But it all kind of goes into the stew of who you are."

Hollywood ending: It has been harder for actress Denise Richards to survive a nasty tabloid spotlight. When she divorced her husband, Charlie Sheen, and soon after was publicly seen being romanced by her best friend's husband, the media emblazoned her with the scarlet letters HS (for husband stealer). "The hardest thing for me," she said, "was trying to be graceful and to have integrity through this whole ordeal. The process of getting divorced is so hard. It should be the other way around. It should be harder to get married—and easier to get a divorce."

In-field out: She divorced three husbands, had an additional five-year romance with Burt Reynolds and now actress Sally Field claims she's finished with relationships. "I'm so way completed; there isn't anybody who would complete me. Change is never easy. You lose your habitual behavior, which allowed you to sort of zone out. You have to be here, you have to be now, and you have to be present." Frequently described as "fierce," Field has a temper, which she displays daily. "If someone treats me with disrespect, I never forget it," she admits. "I have never allowed my heart to be broken." Her friend, Jane Fonda, says "She's strong, extremely smart and capable. You end up saying, 'She's the one who needs to help me.'"

When you're over the hill, that's when you pick up speed. —Quincy Jones

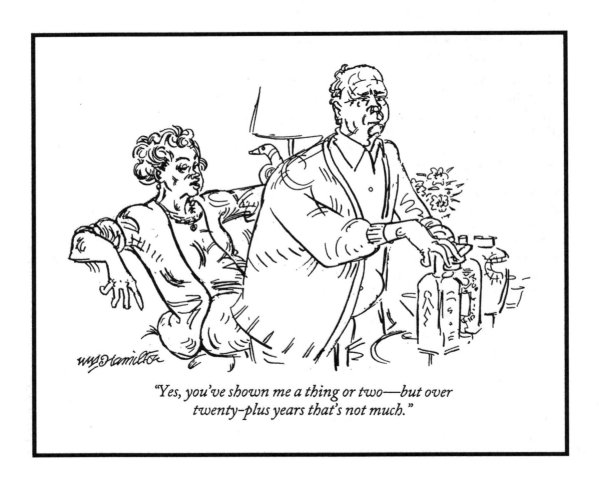

"Yes, you've shown me a thing or two—but over twenty-plus years that's not much."

Quibbling Rivalry—Uninhibited Jealousy

It is stupid to be jealous of your partner's past. That's none of your business. I know that Lisa had sex before we met. I can handle that. Of course, she didn't enjoy it.
—Rich Reynolds

Do you fear me now? Instead of being private in your actions, conversations, and lifestyle, your disappointment becomes so vocal and physical that you terrify the people around you. Struggle to control your temper, which may be temperament that is too old to spank. Don't try irrational behavior to get even.

There's a double standard even today. A man can sleep around and sleep around and nobody asks any questions. But if you're a woman, you make 19 or 20 mistakes, and right away you're a tramp. **—Joan Rivers**

Kelly Osbourne was still an adolescent when her Osbourne family reality TV series invaded her home for edited events in her daily life. Kelly wasn't prepared for the public scrutiny of her every move. Newspaper columnists called her fat. Fashion editors scorned her shoes, her hair, and her makeup. Letters from parents and academics lambasted her for her street language. "My parents were in show business and were used to jealous reviews. But as a teenager, I felt I couldn't do anything right. I had a lot of self-hatred. I just wanted to run away—to disappear into a hole and never come out again." Kelly first hid by taking drugs. Then after hitting rock bottom, she checked into rehab and believes she'll be needing therapy for the rest of her life. "I've paid a stiff price to learn about jealousy—and how never again to be so paranoid."

I gave up dairy, caffeine, and sugar because I was feeling sluggish, tired and anxious. Now I have a lot more energy to feel angry and deprived. **—Jennifer Siegal**

Political retaliation is a double-edged sword that can wound its protagonist. In his presidential election campaign against Dwight D. Eisenhower, Adlai Stevenson needed to diffuse rumors that he was a homosexual because many of his staff were gay. The gossip was untrue, so Stevenson used the line "President Eisenhower and I have a pact. If he'll stop telling lies about me, I'll stop telling the truth about him." While the joke was expertly crafted, it boomeranged because many times the original audience now wanted to know what lies Eisenhower was spreading.

You have to wait ten days to buy a gun in Los Angeles. I can't stay mad that long.
—Emo Philips

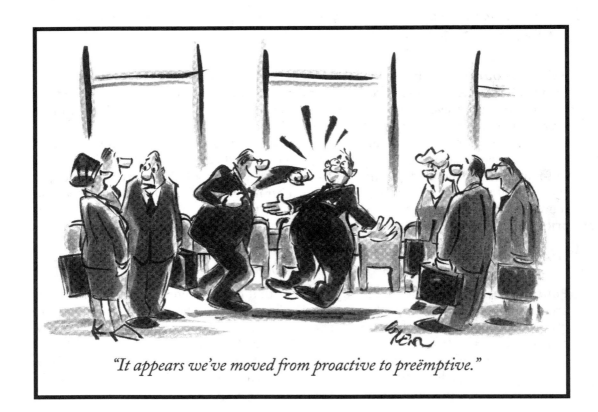

"It appears we've moved from proactive to preëmptive."

Covet Thy Neighbor's Ass—Retaliation

The heaviest load to carry is a grudge.

Blast-off: Long before a female American astronaut tried to whack a rival NASA employee for trying to win a shuttle pilot's affection, murder has been an often-successful strategy for rejection remedy. "In virtually every human society," wrote Daniel Gilbert, "civil and religious law list retaliation and retribution as illegal or immoral—except when they are responses in kind." In other words, a punch thrown second is more legally and morally acceptable than a punch thrown first. But be aware that blind anger can camouflage dangerous potholes in your path. Don't focus so much on the heat of your immediate pain that you forget you'll need a cool head to counter-punch. According to Dr. Dennis Garritan of New York University, "If you are so worked up that you don't feel you can talk then and there, excuse yourself and schedule another meeting for another time." It will give you time to plan your revenge.

Three Hell's Angel motorcyclists—black helmets, swastika flags on their jackets, bodies covered with tattoos, dark glasses—parked their bikes next to a truck and walked into a highway diner. They pushed over a truck driver seated at the counter. One grabbed his sandwich, another drank his coffee and the third bumped him off the chair. After they were all seated, the truck driver didn't say a word, paid the check, and walked out. One of the Hell's Angel cyclists said to the waitress. "He wasn't much of a man, was he?" The waitress looked out the window for a second and said, "No, and he's not much of a truck driver, either. He just backed his truck over three motorcycles."

American Rasputin: Karl Rove, who claims to be the mastermind, if not the ventriloquist, behind George W. Bush, is known for being a maniacal cutthroat political strategist who will use whatever dirty tricks are needed to win. Politics is a no-holds-barred assault on a marble block, according to Rove. "Position the chisel, then hit it hard. Weakness and indecisiveness emboldens your enemies and is an invitation to disaster." He chiseled opponents with "insinuendo," his own term for false rumors, fear, campaign espionage, and ruthless innuendo as weapons, leaving their reputations not just bruised but bloodied. Some say his ruthless divide and conquer strategy has its roots in Rove's youth. At the age of 19, his father walked out on his family to live with gay friends. Then he learned that his father was not his biological parent, and a few years later his mother drove out to the desert, filled the car with carbon monoxide and left a suicide note begging him not to blame himself—a classic assurance that the rejection would make him feel indelibly guilty.

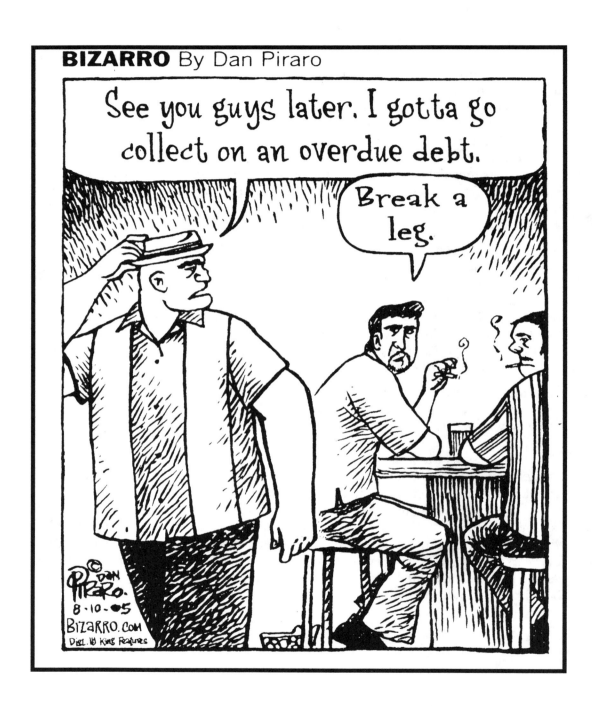

Reach Out and Touch Someone—
A Physical Attack

If you can't beat 'em, arrange to have them beaten. —**George Carlin**

"I'll kill the S.O.B." is generally the first reaction of a major rejection. Good battle cry! Bad remedy! It's an old illusion that somehow we can lift ourselves up through violence. It takes more strength to survive by our wits than it does to beat somebody up. Army commandos and black belt jujitsu experts are taught to kill and maim their enemies. But in private life, they are mild-mannered individuals who will more often back away from a physical confrontation than charge into one.

Never pick a fight with an ugly person. They've got nothing to lose. —**Robin Williams**

The fighting Celtic: There are exceptions, and among the most noteworthy is the confrontation of abusive bullies, not just critics. Gene Tunney, a former world heavyweight boxing champ, was a gentleman novelty in a brutal game. Because he was a scrawny kid at a parochial school in tough Greenwich Village, his nose was often bloodied by gangs on his way home. Finally, his father insisted he put on a pair of boxing gloves and learn to fight. Another example is Red Auerbach, the noted Celtics basketball coach, who had a reputation for being both combative and abrasive. The son of Jewish immigrants, Auerbach was often taunted by opponents' hometown fans. One night, after a torrent of anti-Semitic remarks, a fan assaulted Auerbach as he was leaving the visiting team's locker room. According to a reporter who was present, Auerbach dragged the man back into the locker room and physically bloodied him until the fan, his clothes torn, was hustled away by security. Auerbach calmly rolled down his sleeves, straightened his tie, lit up his victory cigar, and walked confidently to the team bus. After the story appeared in an AP national dispatch, Auerbach rarely heard anti-Semitic remarks again in his 55 years of coaching.

I got into a fight with a really big guy, and he said, "I'm going to mop the floor with your face." I said, "You'll be sorry. You won't be able to get into the corners very well."
—**Emo Philips**

Dr. Steven Carin is president of the American Association of Physician Specialists. But when he was a pre-teen, he was frequently beaten up by bigger kids in his blue-collar inner city neighborhood. His father said "learn to fight or learn how fast you can run." Without much instruction, he began to build his muscles, learning how to avoid punches and, most of all, how to bloody his opponent. As a teenager, he quickly became a gang leader, especially once the other kids found out how quickly he destroyed his attackers. "I know, even today, I can kill a person who physically attacks me. That confidence permits me to first walk away from any confrontation, but if the attack persists, I would throw someone out the window before I would acquiesce." Dr. Carin is my family physician, and you can guess that I always pay his bills immediately.

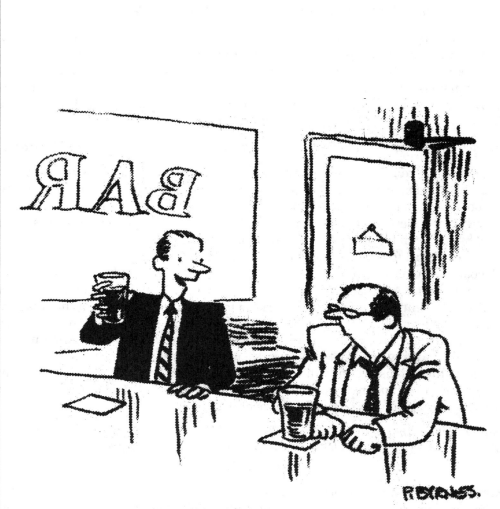

"Ignoring life's lessons is my secret to staying young."

Queen of Denial—Avoiding Controversies

*A friend of mine jogs ten miles a day. If you ever see me running ten miles in a row, tell the friggin' bus driver my arm is still in the door. —**Jeff Shaw***

The path of least resistance: The age of the million-dollar employee lawsuit has caused many business executives who do not have a strong backbone to promote employees who are egotistical, arrogant, pushy, or uncontrollable to another job rather than risk doing something negative that will result in drawn-out controversy. It has now become standard operating procedure and vastly preferable to oil the squeaky wheel by promoting the whacko upward and pass on the problem rather than trying to change or eliminate the bad attitude. Exasperation is not a plan for buying peace and quiet.

Thou shalt not covet they neighbor's house unless they have a well-stocked bar.
*—**W.C. Fields***

How could she do that? Being rejected by a friend is a double sting, because it seems to be so unexpected. Yet the fault lies with you. You presumed too much. Friendship is an elusive, slipper concept, admits William Grimes. It is the neglected first cousin of romantic love, but without a contract or a pledge before God to love, honor, and obey. As long as a common self-indulgent interest continues, friends can impose and presume. In his book *Friendship, An Expose,* Joseph Epstein claims that friendship is an endless series of vexations. He believes that the problem is because no one can precisely define friendship. Is a friend obliged to mortgage his house, donate a kidney or loan a spouse for your two-week vacation? Can't we best avoid disappointments by friends by maintaining a deep gully between obligation and convenience? Samuel Johnson said we take our friends as we find them, not as we would make them. So expect your friend to be a good listener, perhaps even a confessor, but not your self-sacrificing knight.

*The only way to get rid of temptation is to yield to it. —**Oscar Wilde***

Light rights: Jennifer Elison's life with her physician husband was hell on wheels and so was his death. For several years she was belittled, criticized for not acting as a proper doctor's wife and forced to subjugate her feelings of unhappiness. The day after she asked her husband for a divorce, he was killed in an auto accident. Her emotions ran the gamut of bewilderment, sadness, anger and most surprising of all, overwhelming relief. She felt ashamed that she had to hide this relief from family and friends who would surely misunderstand. To be glad that someone is dead is a powerful taboo in our culture. There are also five stages of the grief that can be a straightjacket on how to grieve. "It's never your place to dictate that someone fit your mold on how to grieve," she said. "Family members must be forgiven if they are pleased to be getting their lives back."

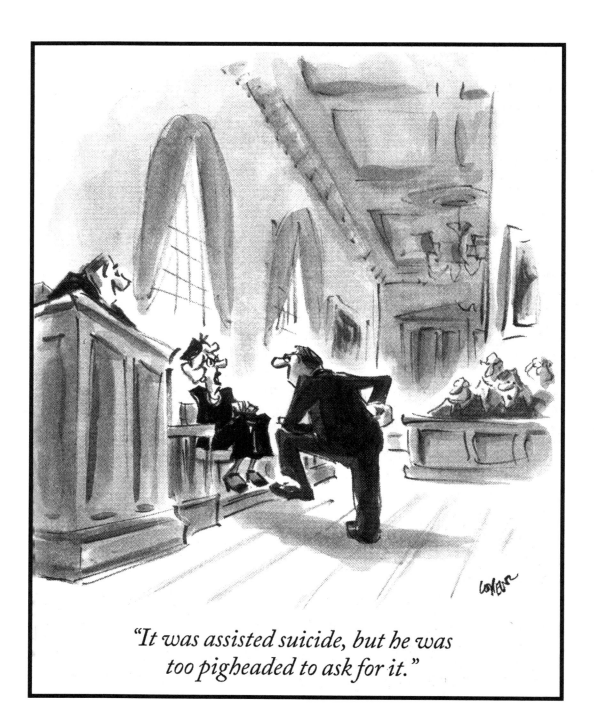

"It was assisted suicide, but he was
too pigheaded to ask for it."

A Grave Responsibility—
Joining Murderer's Row

I made a killing in the stock market. My broker lost all my money, so I killed him.
—Jim Loy

Getting whacked: Whether it's called murder, assassination, or just taking somebody out, revenge murders are on the rise and so are foreign assassinations. Fifteen American presidents have been the object of assassination attempts and four—Lincoln, Garfield, McKinley and Kennedy—were successful (or unsuccessful depending on your political persuasion). And America has often been accused of helping foment the assassination of foreign leaders.

I asked my father, "Do you think a family should have the right to withdraw life support on a loved one?" And he said, "It depends on which kid." —Hugh Fink

"I'm going to kill that s.o.b." has become so automatic and an oath when you feel wronged, no one calls 911 to report a potential assassin at bay. In recent years, committing murder without prosecution has been the synopsis of so many *Sopranos* episodes and *Terminator* films that many adolescents grow to adulthood before they learn it's against the law. And Iraq's suicide bombers have added a new dimension—martyrdom—to the popularity of murder without exit. In England, a 31-year-old loner was told by his married lover that she wouldn't leave her husband for him, so he beat her to death with a mallet. Five years later, when his teenage girlfriend also rejected him, he killed her by torching her house. You don't expect every rejected lover to be a psychopath. But the moral of this grisly report is that handing out a rejection notice is no trivial scenario and should be finessed even before the play starts. Loneliness can be sad, but rejection can kill.

A woman asked the pharmacist for some arsenic. "What do you want it for?" he asked. "I want to give it to my husband," she answered. "You can't do that, you'll kill him and I'll lose my license." The woman showed him a photograph of her husband in bed with the pharmacist's wife. "Oh," he said, "I didn't know you had a prescription."

Grapes of wrath: Fiction writers and poets are a Rabelaisian esprit de corps when it comes to abusing obstreperous critics. They kill them off in their literature. James Merrill, an established American poet, became annoyed with taunting critics who downgraded his comic work because he was an admitted homosexual. So he named his fictional characters with the names of live critics and provided a range of ugly death scenarios about them in his most heralded works. He claims that their criticism either ceased or immediately became more scholarly.

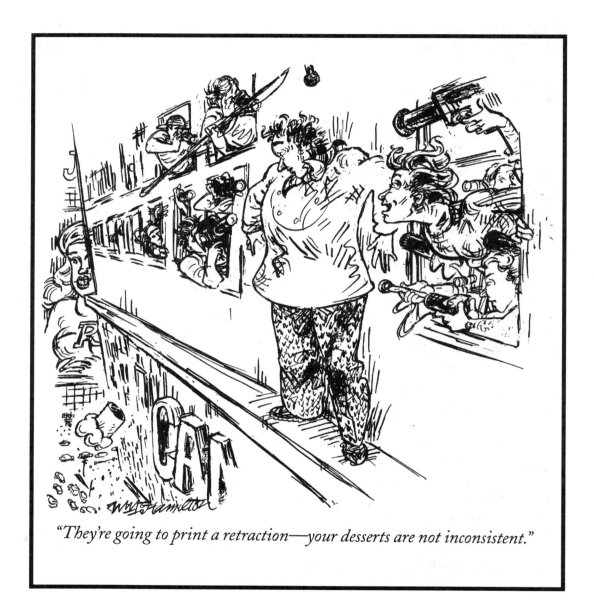

"They're going to print a retraction—your desserts are not inconsistent."

Dead Wrong—Contemplating Suicide

Did you ever go out on a date, because you were too lazy to commit suicide?
—Judy Tenuta

The ultimate rejection: As abhorrent as suicide may appear as a serious consequence of rejection and depression, it is becoming increasingly more frequent as a single benefit option. Some call suicide a blind escape for selfish people because it is does more harm (a living death) to those who are closely related. But depression is a real disease that results from a chemical imbalance. In the 1970's, when Tony Bennett, whom Frank Sinatra called "the best singer in the business," felt he was washed up—he couldn't get a manager or a record deal, and was beset by financial, drug, and marital problems, contemplating suicide as his only "out." He turned to his son, who cannily repositioned Bennett's style to MTV hipsters, and his career suddenly turned upward and has stayed that way for thirty years. "I've had so many graduations from the school of hard knocks, you wouldn't believe," said Bennett.

You might be lonely, miserable, depressed and suicidal, but none of that matters—as long as you're happy.—Don Haupman

Your number's up: According to the National Mental Health Association more than 30,000 people in the U.S. committed suicide in 2001, and rejection or failure was the highest percentage cause. With teens, aged 12 to 17, suicide is a recurrent theme. In 2000, three million youths seriously contemplated suicide. One-third of that group actually attempted suicide, and the rate is increasing, according to the 2003 Youth Risk Survey by the Ohio Department of Health. One of every 12 U.S. college students has made a suicide plan, so it is a rare college that has not established a counseling and prevention department. Their responsibility is to educate parents as well as students about the possible risks associated with the depression that result from adolescent trauma.

The FDA approved the first-ever transdermal patch for the treatment of depression. Simply remove the backing and press the patch firmly over your mother's mouth.
—Tina Fey

Snap, crackle, and plop: Female suicide incidents are most frequent when a marriage is dissolved. Photographer Dina Arbus was famous for pictures of deviants that "nobody else would see." But after the breakup of her marriage, she went into the depth of alienation. "My work doesn't do it for me anymore." Eventually her depression became self-loathing. She was discovered lying in an empty bathtub with her wrists slit. Female suicide is one of the most frequent endings of many dark cinema plots. And its effect is mind-boggling and long lasting. Progressive female critics decried the dual side-by-side suicide solution in the film *Thelma & Louise* as not being a positive alternative choice for women in trouble with the law.

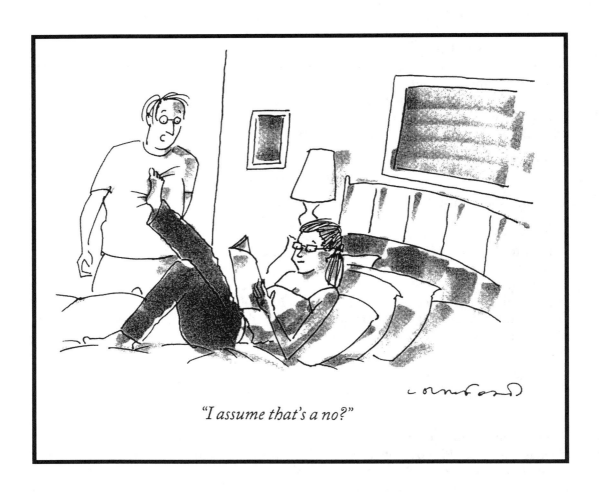

"I assume that's a no?"

Four Big Benefits—
Rejection Can Be a Blessing

"What's the meaning of rejection?" Philosopher Julian Baggini, is his book *What's It All About,* claims, "Change, through rejection, is the pith and marrow of life, together with the responsibility of selecting values we wish to live by. Change is necessary for growth, and there is a library of examples of how an initial rejection turned out to be a blessing."

I have a Dreamgirl: After Jennifer Hudson was eliminated in an early round of *American Idol,* Simon Cowell, one of the regular judges, told Hudson, "You're out of your depth in this one. You only get one chance at it, and the people who don't win will never be seen again." Hudson was devastated, and for three years no matter what audition she tried, Simon's hard-hitting rejection trumped her confidence. Then one day she was asked to be one of 784 women tested for the part of Effie White in the movie version of the Broadway musical *Dreamgirls*. Effie had a fabulous voice and vast ambition, but also was a diva with a chip on her shoulder who went into a tailspin when she was pushed aside and then fired from the Supremes-like trio she had helped found. When it came time to be tested, Hudson felt her life so mirrored the character's life that her emotional reading and singing wowed the casting team. "I know it's unbelievable. I would end up being grateful for one of the most humiliating rejections in my life," she reported, "but nobody could do that part better than me because I lived it." Film critics agreed. Jennifer Hudson's Oscar-winning performance became the most memorable in the movie.

If you think of rejection as a temporary setback, it can provide at least four opportunities to turn failure into success:

(1) The freedom to fail is as much a part of the American dream as life, liberty and the pursuit of women,

(2) The opportunity to redefine yourself, to do your own thing, like start a business because you got fired, or change your life style because you got divorced, or rephotograph your life's story without totally fabricating your resume,

(3) Retire, not from something but to something. Cash in the reward you've earned that's more than a Social Security check,

(4) Win public sympathy that can jump-start your flagging career.

To each of us, at certain points in our lives, there come opportunities to rearrange our formulas and assumptions—not necessarily to be rid of the old, but to profit by adding something new. **—Leo Buscaglia**

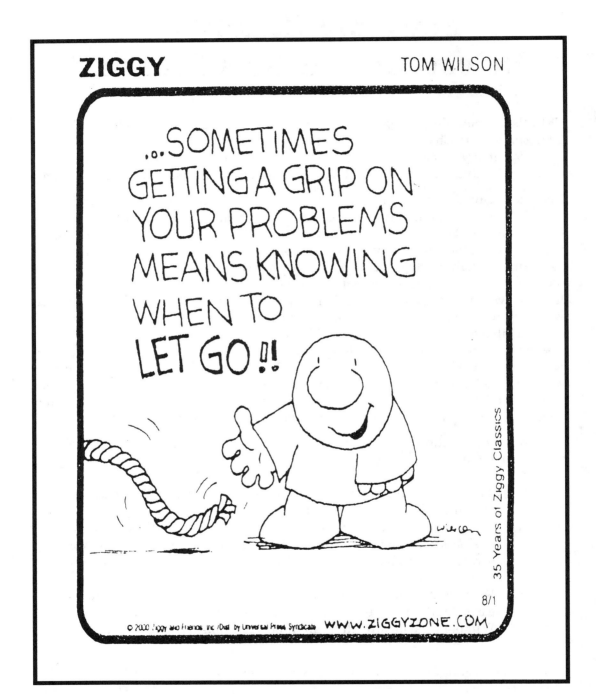

The Unconventional Man—
The Freedom to Fail

In many ways, rejection was the best thing that happened to me. —**Abraham Lincoln**

Win, lose, or draw: Being able to try something—win, lose or draw—is a privilege. Failure begets wisdom, and college students pay a lot to get it. Think of the fear of failure as a surface injury—a temporary distraction. Winston Churchill turned to politics because he twice failed the entrance exams to the Royal Military Academy at Sandhurst.

Failure is a fiction cleverly disguised as a disappointment. —**Richard Carlson**

Not on TV: How does one move on when you've tried and failed over and over to reach some unattainable goal that's just beyond your ability, such as a medical certification or law bar exam? The only one who remembers such a failure is you, unless you happen to strike out with the bases loaded in a World Series game. Don't keep harping on it, unless you're just begging for sympathy.

Rush Limbaugh flunked out of Southeast Missouri State University in his freshman year, and ever since he's felt complimented whenever anybody said his work was sophomoric.

Change of direction: Start by re-evaluating the event. Be realistic, not habitually optimistic. At some point, you need to banish doubt and despair. A mistake is not a failure. Wordsworth's "Dejection: An Ode" celebrates joy as an audaciously unashamed locution "to be happy." It is something to "animate and ennoble ourselves," said Mathew Arnold.

You're perverted, twisted, and sick. I like that in a person.

Dig this: Politicians use this story to show that benefits can come from spreading dirt.

One day a donkey fell into a well and couldn't get out. The farmer worried that the donkey would die and smell up the neighborhood, so he called all his friends to come over and help him bury the animal in the well. All of them started to throw dirt down the well, but after each spade full, the donkey would shake off the dirt and take a step up over the packed dirt. Eventually, the dirt became so high that the donkey was able to step over the edge of the well to safety.

First class rage: When Mahatma Gandhi was a young lawyer, he was tossed off a train in South Africa because he was a nonwhite man riding in a first-class compartment. His rage at the rejection was so strong that Gandhi made up his mind at that moment: he would go into politics to stand up for the rights of his race no matter the cost.

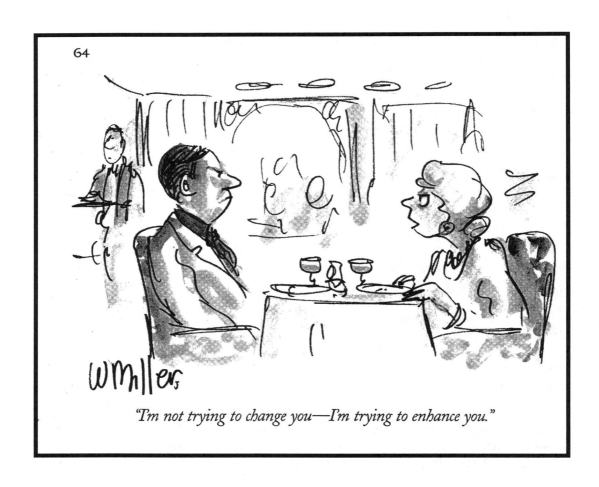

"I'm not trying to change you—I'm trying to enhance you."

A Swift Kick in the Career—
Starting Your Own Thing

My boss got kicked upstairs. You'll find him on the roof.

Home of the brave: Even though the odds against success are daunting—only one start-up in ten lasts longer than three years—there have been few stronger incentives for many of America's most successful entrepreneurs than the day they were cast loose from a job they were holding. First, their despair was overwhelming. With debts to pay and families to raise, they not only felt unappreciated by the human race, they felt rejected. The initial instinct was to look for another job. When that stalled, more than 1,000 per day set out to prove that the world may not be flat, but it was certainly wrong. They raised money to start their own business, and their success became the legend of the American dream. It is possible.

The story of my success is that after a hundred failures to produce electric lighting, I said, "I have not failed. I just discovered 100 ways not to invent the light bulb."
—Thomas Edison

Land of the fee: After nearly 20 years as an executive with the American Medical Association and the National Cancer Institute, Donna Grande's job was terminated as a result of budget cuts. So she decided to start her own consulting business and be available for everyone in the health field—for a fee. As an avid scuba diver, she knew that careful preparation is needed before plunging into an unknown sea which you can only hope won't be shark infested. With mask, fins, and a tank full of air, she jumped off her boat with both feet into her new adventure. She was lucky. She had a husband with website skills and a neighbor who was a graphic designer. She was quickly able to offer her clients program development in charting the seas between public health/medicine and public/private interests. She is doing swimmingly well.

*Glory is fleeting, but obscurity is forever. —**Napoleon***

The first centerfold: As a teen-ager, he couldn't jitterbug and he didn't know how to dress, so Hugh Hefner was dumped by his childhood sweetheart. She found another man and married him. The he got fired by *Esquire* magazine for demanding a $5 raise. So, Hefner decided to reinvent himself. He started to refer to himself as Hef instead of Hugh and took up dancing lessons. A few years later, he decided to become a womanizer and invented *Playboy* magazine.

*Once upon a time, a handsome prince asked a beautiful princess to marry him. She said, "No!" After he was rejected, the prince thought a great deal about the meaning of life, and now he is living happily ever after by going fishing, hunting, playing golf, drinking beer and farting whenever he wants. —**Bill Carbone***

Bad student loan: The most common career rejection starts in college. Mario Batali, TV star-chef of New York's most famous Italian restaurant, was bounced from Rutgers as an international banking major, so he went to a London cooking school. "I still have nightmares that I passed the college exams and became a fucking loan clerk."

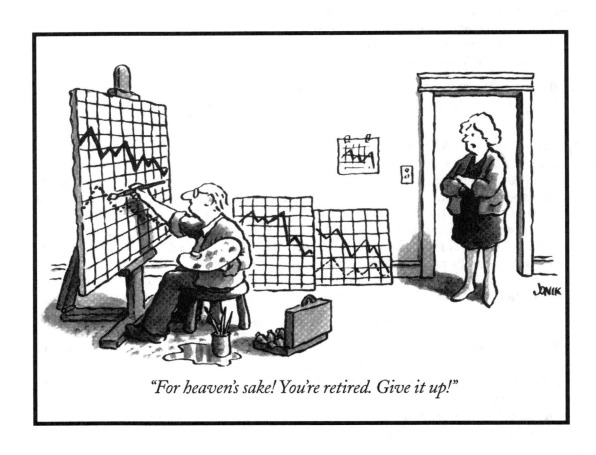

"For heaven's sake! You're retired. Give it up!"

Too Good to be Through—
Retiring to Something

You know it's time to retire when you wake up with morning-after taste in your mouth and you know darn well you didn't do anything the night before. —**Hal Scholle**

There is a time to retire. Unless they are required to retire at age 62 or 65, the age that Social Security benefits kick in, most executives in Fortune 500 companies resist going quietly into the night as long as they can. In our book *It's Never Too Late to Plant a Tree: Your Guide to Never Retiring,* Morrie Helitzer and I put the spotlight on 65 seniors who have not only accepted retirement with grace but went on to inspirational projects that benefited not only themselves but their families, their communities, and even their nation.

I want to live to be a hundred years old, because you rarely read obituaries about people over a hundred. —**George Burns**

Ageism: Today millions, who originally answered "Anything I want to," when asked what they were planning to do when they retire, are finding that capricious retirement is less than fulfilling. They feel they still have much to contribute. Bobbie Battista was one of CNN's original anchors, but left with a buyout package after 23 years. It was an amount of cash she needed to start her own public relations business advising companies on how to navigate the media world. In only four years she exceeded the $100,000 salary mark that she had with CNN. Her advice is that you've got to balance your aspirations with reality. "Ageism," a social disease based upon discrimination against senior citizens, is a prejudice that is hard to defeat, claim columnists Humberto and Georgina Cruz, and a chronic illness could prevent or limit many lines of work. "But don't take your first rejection as a final opinion. Explore options and start again."

Older and wiser: Here are ten keys to successful aging, accorded to the National Institute on Aging at the University of Pittsburgh: (1) build a network of close friends and family, (2) enjoy hobbies, (3) be optimistic, (4) exercise, (5) sleep seven to eight hours a night, (6) don't smoke, (7) eat more fruits and vegetables, (8) get enough calcium and vitamin D through low-dairy products, (9) take common sense precautions like seat belts, sunscreen, flossing teeth and limiting alcoholic beverages, and (10) get recommended health screenings and annual flu shots. Moving to the Sun Belt is no guarantee of a happy retirement. This is where more and more unhappy seniors can be found killing time watching TV or helping Indian casinos gamble away their savings. Retirement can give a person a fresh chance at happiness—or present some dangerous alternatives.

When he retired he became a discount exterminator. He'd come over with a rolled-up magazine.

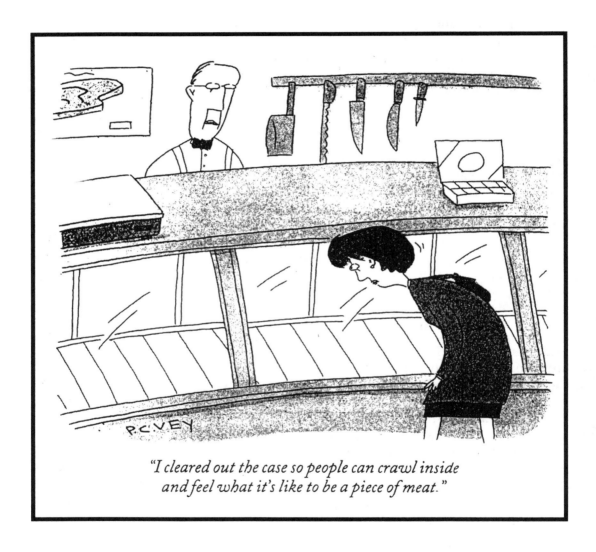

"*I cleared out the case so people can crawl inside
and feel what it's like to be a piece of meat.*"

A Star is Born—Getting Public Sympathy

The Debbie Reynolds Syndrome: Even if you're not in the public eye, the sympathy generated by a dramatic rejection can eventually become a positive force for good. It's called the Debbie Reynolds syndrome. As a young actress Reynolds was dumped by her husband, singer Eddie Fisher, who fell in love with and eventually married Elizabeth Taylor. The public outrage, fanned by the ominous drum roll of gossipy supermarket tabloids, had a longer run than any Broadway musical. Suddenly, the public wanted to know all about Debbie, rushed to her B pictures which became financial bonanzas, and for years the name "Debbie" was one of the most popular names given to newborn girls.

My boy, Bill: More recently, Hillary Clinton was the unexpected beneficiary of glowing coverage during the Monica Lewinsky fracas. According to Joshua Green, "As the wronged but dignified spouse, Clinton's favorable ratings soared. This must have been a disquieting experience, because she now found herself rehabilitated for reasons that had nothing to do with her brains or talent." She used this popularity to help ride off to the U.S. Senate and become a candidate for President.

Last week, Monica Lewinsky celebrated her 31st birthday. My, how time flies. It seems like only yesterday she was crawling around the Oval Office on her hands and knees.
—Jay Leno

Die Ana: It was public sympathy that encouraged an energetic Princess Diana to feast as a globe-trotting humanitarian on front pages for several years after her divorce from Prince Charles. Her tragic death produced one of England's largest periods of mourning.

Sordid photos: Vanessa Williams was a phenomenon. She was the first black Miss America, but the first to lose her title when nude photographs of her in a compromising position ran in *Penthouse*. The public was so incensed by this trifling reason for her disqualification that combined with her talent for acting and singing, she became one of the most famous Miss Americas of all time. "Don't try to please. Don't try to be nice," she said. "Be strong enough to voice your opinion; just don't try to grow up too fast."

I've learned we are always responsible for what we do, unless we are celebrities.
—Adrienne Helitzer

The moral of these stories is that rejection can be used as a steppingstone in business as well as your personal life. Instead of hiding it, reach for sympathy from friends and, most often, the public. For this strategy to work, you'll need something for your supporters to buy—a product or a service—and public relations specialists to guide you.

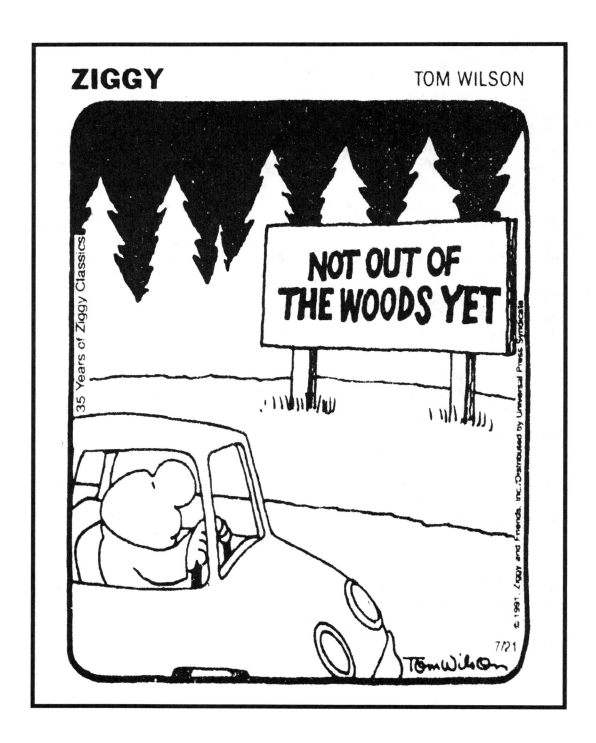

The Last Word

A death-defying act: Skeptics frequently challenge me that "Humor is just a diversion. It's not practical at momentous occasions—like terminal illness and death." Quite the contrary! I am often asked to speak at memorial services of close friends and relatives. Each time, I draft a few humorous anecdotes that I remember sharing with the deceased and then ask the family for permission to use them. Most often they not only give their approval but add, "Oh, we've got better ones than those," and proceed to give me hilarious stories that meant the most to them. And when I use them in my eulogy, I feel a warming breeze float over the audience that helps them, as they laugh, to rediscover the humanity and love of the deceased. It works every time.

A few years ago, a friend of mine who had a terminal illness took the time, before he died, to write a personal letter to each of his children. In each, besides some personal advice, he recollected one funny incident that he had shared and how much their long, intimate talks meant to him. The letters were read and reread and each became a family heirloom. He wrote, "Even though I may not be here, we can still continue to talk together as long as you wish. Every time you do some goofball thing that temporarily turns your world into a slapstick comedy, say 'Dad would have loved this.' Then tell me about it. And whenever you have a problem and you're seeking a solution, ask yourself 'What would Dad do?' And even though you're all alone, don't be afraid to speak out loud. You talk. I'll listen."

When you walk through a storm,
Hold your head up high
And don't be afraid of the dark.
At the end of the storm is a golden sky
And the sweet silver song of a lark.
Walk on through the wind
Walk on through the rain
Tho' your dreams be tossed and blown.
Walk on, walk on with hope in your heart
And you'll never walk alone.
You'll never walk alone.

—Rogers and Hammerstein
Carousel

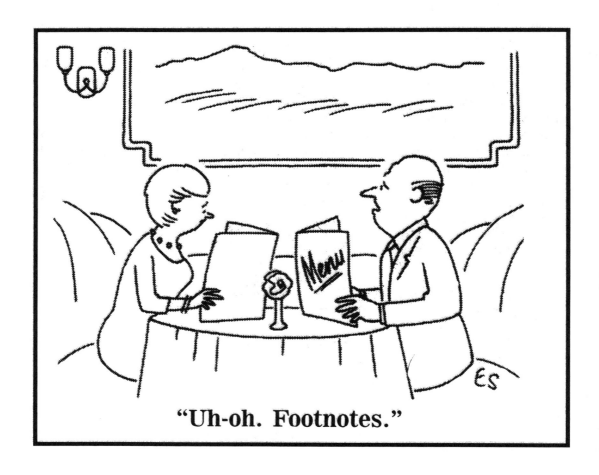

"Uh-oh. Footnotes."

References

Angier, Natalie. *"Almost Before We Spoke, We Swore."* New York Times 20 September 2005.

Asher, Steven R. and John D. Coie. *Peer Rejection in Childhood*. Cambridge, UK: Cambridge UP, 1990.

Bierman, Karen L. *Peer Rejection*. New York: Guilford Press, 2004.

Booher, Dianna Daniels. *Making Friends with Yourself and Other Strangers,* New York: Julian Messner, 1982.

Braiker, Harriet B. *The Disease to Please, Curing the People-Pleasing Syndrome,* New York: McGraw-Hill, 2005.

Brown, Judy. *Comedy Thesaurus*. Philadelphia: Quirk Books, 2005.

Buckingham, Marcus and Donald O. Clifton. *Now, Discover Your Strengths*. New York: Free Press, 2001.

Canfield, Jack and Mark Victor Hansen. *Chicken Soup for the Soul*. Deerfield Beach, FL: Health Communications, Inc., 1993.

Carlson, Richard. *Easier Than You Think*. San Francisco: Harper, 2005.

Carlson, Richard. *What About the Big Stuff*. New York: Hyperion, 2002.

Carnegie, Dale. *How to Win Friends and Influence People,* New York, Pocket Books, 1990 edition.

Cini, Joanne. *Kingmaker: Be the One Your Company Wants to Keep*. New York: Prentice Hall, 2004.

Fisher, Roger. *Getting to Yes: Negotiating Agreement Without Giving In*. Boston: Houghton-Mifflin, 1991.

Foreman, George. *Guide to Life*. Simon and Schuster: New York, 2002,

Frank, Carol. *Do As I Say, Not As I Did!* Dallas: Brown Books, 2005.

Fuhrman, John. *Reject Me—I Love It*. Hummelstown, PA: Success Publishers, 1997.

Gilbert, Daniel. *Stumbling on Happiness*. Boston: Harvard University, 2006.

Green, Joey. *The Road to Success Is Paved with Failure*. New York: Time Warner, 2001.

Guthrie, Nancy, *Holding on to Hope*. Wheaton, IL: Tyndale House Publishers, 2002.

Halberstam, Joshua. *Everyday Ethics*. New York: Penguin Books, 1993.

Helitzer, Mel. *The Dream Job: Sports Publicity, Promotion and Marketing*. Athens, OH: University Sports Press, 2004.

Helitzer, Mel and Morrie Helitzer. *It's Never Too Late to Plant a Tree: Your Guide to Never Retiring*. Athens, OH: University Sports Press, 2004.

Helitzer, Mel and Mark Shatz. *Comedy Writing Secrets*. Cincinnati, OH: Writer's Digest, 2005.

Hitti, Miranda. *Dancing Your Way to Better Health*. WebMD Feature, July 7, 2005.

Jaffe, Azriela. *Starting From 'No'—10 Strategies to Overcome Fear of Rejection and Succeed in Business*. Chicago, IL: Dearborn Publishing, 1999.

Jeffers, Susan. *Feel the Fear and Do It Anyway*. San Diego: Harcourt Brace Jovanovich, 1987.

Johnson, Spencer. *Who Moved My Cheese?* New York: G.P. Putnam & Sons, 1998.

Kabat-Zinn, Jon. *Wherever You Go, There You Are*. New York: Hyperion, 1994.

Klein, Allen. *The Healing Power of Humor*. Los Angeles: Jeremy P. Tarcher: 1989.

Kushner, Harold S. *How Good Do We Have to Be? A New Understanding of Guilt and Forgiveness*. Thorndike, ME: G.K. Hall, 1997.

Lappe, Frances Moore and Jeffrey Perkins. *You Have the Power*. New York: Jeremy P. Tarcher/Penguin, 2004.

Lunden, Joan, and Andrea Cagan. *A Bend in the Road Is Not the End of the Road*. New York: William Morrow & Company, 1998.

McCullough, Michael E., Steven J. Sandage, and Everett L. Worthington, Jr. *To Forgive Is Human: How to Put Your Past in the Past*. Downers Grove, IL: Intervarsity Press, 1997.

McGinnis, Alan Loy. *The Friendship Factor*. Minneapolis: Augsburg Books, 2004.

Moe, Barbara. *Coping with Rejection*. New York: Rosen Publishing Group, 2001.

Mortell, Art. *The Courage to Fail*. New York: McGraw-Hill, 1992.

Pearson, Judy C. and Paul E. Nelson, *An Introduction to Human Communication*. New York: McGraw-Hill, 2000, 2005.

Pennebaker, James W. *Opening Up: The Healing Power of Confiding in Others.* , New York: William Morrow and Company, 1990.

Potter-Efron, Ron and Pat Potter-Efron. *Letting Go of Anger: The 10 Most Common Anger Styles and What to Do About Them*. Oakland: New Harbinger Publications, 2005.

Preston, John. *Complete Idiot's Guide to Managing Your Moods,* New York: Alpha Publishing House, 2006.

Richman, Linda. *I'd Rather Laugh*. New York: Warner Books, 2001.

Robbins, Anthony. *Awaken the Giant Within*. New York: Simon & Schuster, 1991.

Robbins, Anthony. *Notes From a Friend*. New York: Simon & Schuster, 1995.

Rogers, Fred. *The World According to Mister Rogers*. New York: Hyperion, 2003.

Rogers, Fred. *You Are Special*. New York: Penguin Books, 1994.

Salerno, Steve. *Sham*. New York: Crown Publishers, 2005.

Sark. *Change Your Life Without Getting Out of Bed*. New York: Simon & Schuster, 1999.

Savage, Elayne. *Don't Take It Personally: The Art of Dealing with Rejection*. Oakland: New Harbinger Publications, 1997.

Scholle, Hal. *Getting Older*. Naperville, IL: River Bend Press, 1998.

Sellers, Heather. *Page After Page*. Cincinnati, OH: Writer's Digest Books, 2005.

Selzer, Steven Michael. *Life's Little Relaxation Book*. New York: Three Rivers Press, 2005.

Shellenbarger, Sue. "Work and Family: The Latest Rules on What Not to Talk About." *The Wall Street Journal* 21 July 2005.

Siegel, Dr. Bernie S. *101 Exercises for the Soul*. Novato, CA: New World Library, 2005.

Stoddard, Alexandra. *The Art of the Possible*. New York: William Morrow and Company, 1995.

Stout, Hilary. "Family Matters," *The Wall Street Journal* 7 July 2005.

Talen, Bill. *What Should I Do If Reverend Billy Is In My Store?* New York: New Press, 2003.

Telushkin, Joseph. *Words That Hurt, Words That Heal*. New York: William Morrow, 1996.

Tucker, Tanya. *100 Ways to Beat the Blues*. New York: Simon & Schuster, 2005.

Vanzant, Iyania. *Yesterday, I Cried*. New York: Simon & Schuster, 1998.

Walker, Laura Jensen. *Through the Rocky Road and into the Rainbow Sherbet*. Grand Rapids, MI: Baker Book House, 2002.

Wallin, Pauline. *Taming Your Inner Brat: A Guide for Transforming Self-Defeating Behavior*. Camp Hill, PA: 2005.

"Interpersonal Rejection"—Godwin, Oxford University Press, New York, 10016, 2005.

"Overcoming Rejection"—Hammond, Impact Publishers, Inc., Atascadero, CA, 93423

Recommended Reading

*Anatomy of an Illness—***Norman Cousins**
*Conquering Anxiety and Depression Through Exercise—***Keith Johngard**
*Cursing in America—***Timothy B. Jay**
*Everybody Wants Your Money—***David W. Latko**
*Friendship: An Expose—***Joseph Epstein**
*Get Out of Your Mind and Into Your Life—***Steven Hayes**
*Get Organized Now—***Marcia Garcia**
*It Takes a Village—***Hillary Clinton**
*Never Good Enough—***Monica Ramirez Basco**
*Looney Laws and Silly Statues—***Sheryl Lindsell-Roberts**
*Love and Respect—***Emerson Eggerich**
*Master Your Fears—***Linda Sapadin**
*The Art of Civilized Conversation—***Margaret Shepherd**
*The Discomfort Zone—***Jonathan Frazen**
*The Lazy Husband—***Josh Coleman**
*The Mars of Venus Diet and Exercise Solution—***John Gray**
*The Primal Scream—***Arthur Janov**
*The Rejected Collection—***Matthew Diffee**
*The Road Less Traveled—***M. Scott Peck**
*The Tibetan Book of Living and Dying—***Sogyal Dinpoche**
*Tough Choices—***Carly Fiorina**
*Should I Stay or Go—***Lee Raffel**
*Perfectly Perfect—***Martha Stewart**
*What's It All About—***Julian Baggini**
*You Don't Have to Suffer—***Judy Tatelbaum**